The Planter's Guide, and Family Book of Medicine;
for the Instruction and Use of Planters, Families,
Country People, and All Others Who May Be Out of
the Reach of Physicians, or Unable to Employ Them.

The Planter's Guide, and Family Book of Medicine;

for the Instruction and Use of
Planters, Families, Country People,
and All Others Who May Be Out of
the Reach of Physicians, or Unable
to Employ Them.

J. Hume Simons

With Particular Directions Respecting Asiatic Cholera,
by a Charleston Physician.

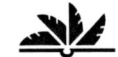

THE UNIVERSITY OF SOUTH CAROLINA PRESS

*An AccessAble Book, Published in Cooperation with
University Libraries, University of South Carolina*

Cloth edition of *The Planter's Guide and Family Book of Medicine for the Instruction and Use of Planters, Families, Country People, and All Others Who May Be Out of the Reach of Physicians, or Unable to Employ Them* published by M'Carter & Allen, Charleston, South Carolina, 1848

Paperback edition published by
the University of South Carolina Press,
Columbia, South Carolina 29208

www.sc.edu/uscpress

Manufactured in the United States of America

20 19 18 17 16 15 14 13 12 11
10 9 8 7 6 5 4 3 2 1

Library of Congress Cataloging-in-Publication data is available.

ISBN 978-1-57003-930-0 (pbk)

THE

PLANTER'S GUIDE,

AND

FAMILY BOOK OF MEDICINE;

FOR THE INSTRUCTION AND USE OF

PLANTERS, FAMILIES, COUNTRY PEOPLE,

AND ALL OTHERS WHO MAY BE OUT OF THE REACH OF
PHYSICIANS, OR UNABLE TO EMPLOY THEM.

By J. HUME SIMONS, M. D.

WITH

PARTICULAR DIRECTIONS RESPECTING ASIATIC CHOLERA,

BY A CHARLESTON PHYSICIAN.

CHARLESTON, S. C.:
M'CARTER & ALLEN.
COLUMBIA:—ALLEN, M'CARTER, & CO.

PREFACE.

THE flattering success which has attended the publication of the first and second editions of the "Family Medicine," has induced the issue of a stereotype edition, which is now offered to the public, carefully revised, and with the few typographical inaccuracies corrected. The work has been submitted to the scrutiny of some of the most eminent physicians in the United States, and received their approval; and the author flatters himself that the treatment which he recommends is in accordance with the practice of the most enlightened physicians of the age.

For the arrangement of the Medical Table he claims entire originality, as well as for the arrangement of the whole work, which has been condensed as much as possible, to avoid verbosity, and to collect the most useful matter into the smallest space.

With entire confidence, then, in the correctness, accuracy, and utility of this work, and the assurance that it is no hasty production, but the result of years of labor and research, it is again offered to the public.

INDEX.

1*

. READ THESE REMARKS AND DIRECTIONS CAREFULLY.

. THE doses set down in the Table of Medicines may be considered as suitable to the *generality* of constitutions. But it must be borne in mind, that *all* persons do not require the *same* dose. You must, therefore, use your judgment, to increase or lessen a dose from the quantity set down in the Table of Medicines, according to circumstances, the age, constitution of the patient, &c. Bear in mind, moreover, that you are not *always* to give a dose as many times as the Table of Medicines directs; but that these directions are to be considered as instructing you *how often* a dose *can* be given during the day or night. Sometimes it is only necessary to give a dose once a day or night; or if it is given two or three times, to divide the dose into as many smaller doses. You will observe, also, that the *same* medicine is sometimes set down in different parts of the Table, under different heads, and in different doses. For instance, when Calomel is to be given as a Cathartic (or purge), the dose must be larger than when it is to be given as an Alterative. If, therefore, you wish to give it as a Cathartic (or purge), look for it under the head of Cathartics, in the Table of Medicines, and give the dose set down there. But if you wish to use it as an Alterative, look for it under the head of Alteratives, and give the dose directed there. Follow the same directions in giving Emetics, Stimulants, Tonics, or any of the others.

If you wish to find a medicine, and you know it to be a Cathartic, Emetic, or any other, look in the Table of Medicines which is arranged alphabetically, under the heads of Cathartics, Emetics, &c. If not, and you know the name, look in the Index, and you will find it under the letter with which the name begins. Do the same in looking for any disease, poultice, plaster, &c.

If you go to see a person taken ill, examine the symptoms, that is to say, feel the pulse, the skin, look at the tongue, and ask the patient, or those who were with him before and when he was taken, to tell you all that has happened ; if the patient has been purging or puking, where the pains are, &c. Always ask if the bowels are free, for if not they must be opened, as a general rule. Feel the patient's pulse, just as you get into the room, and then feel your own ; the taller a person is, the slower the pulse, as a general rule. Feel the pulse again after a little while, for a patient is apt to be excited, or alarmed, by any one coming in suddenly, and so you may be deceived by his pulse. Practise with your own pulse, feeling it frequently on getting up in the morning, after walking or eating, &c., and you can soon learn to distinguish between a sick and a well person by the pulse. For the pulse is the best index we have of sickness or health. The tongue can not always be depended upon, for some persons have habitually foul, and others clean tongues.

Lastly, examine your patient very carefully ; if he has a fever, learn all his symptoms and pains, and where they are, &c., then look among the fevers until you find one in which his symptoms correspond with those in the book ; then treat him accordingly. Do the same with all the other diseases.

A TABLE OF THE PRINCIPAL MEDICINES

USED IN THE TREATMENT OF MEDICAL DISEASES, ARRANGED IN ALPHABETICAL ORDER, ACCORDING TO THEIR PROPERTIES, WITH THE DOSES ADAPTED TO THE AGE OF THE PATIENT.

ANTISPASMODICS, or such Medicines as relieve Cramps and disorders attended with contractions and convulsive movements of the body or limbs.

	FOR A GROWN PERSON.	FOR A CHILD FROM 5 TO 7 YEARS OF AGE.	HOW MANY TIMES A DAY.	IN WHAT TO BE TAKEN.
ASAFŒTIDA. Dose:				
Of the tincture,	25 to 60 drops.	10 to 15 drops.	Every 3 or 4 hours.	In a little water.
In pills,	8 to 12 grains.	3 to 4 grains.	2 or 3 times a day.	Rolled in the fingers.
Of the volatile spirit,	15 to 30 drops.	3 to 5 drops.	Every 3 or 4 hours.	In a little water.
Good for fainting, weak stomach, low spirits, nervous complaints, hysterics, pain in the bowels, coughs.				
AMBER—of the rectified oil. Dose:	7 to 8 drops.	2 to 3 drops.	2 or 3 times a day.	In a little syrup.
For coughs and nervous feelings.				
ÆTHER—Sulphuric compound Spirits:	40 to 50 drops.	6 to 8 drops.	2 or 3 times a day.	In a little water.
For cramps, wind in the bowels, and asthma.				
AMMONIA, or Hartshorn. Dose:	20 to 40 drops.	2 to 3 drops.	2 or 3 times a day.	In a little water.
For fainting and low spirits.				

2

ANTISPASMODICS.—Continued.

	FOR A GROWN PERSON.	FOR A CHILD FROM 5 TO 7 YEARS OF AGE.	HOW MANY TIMES A DAY.	IN WHAT TO BE TAKEN.
CAMPHOR — of the gum in pills. Dose:	3 to 4 grains.	1 to 2 grains.	2 or 3 times a day.	Rolled between the fingers.
Of the spirits, Of the julep,	3 to 4 tablespoonfuls	2 to 3 teaspoonfuls.	3 or 4 times a day.	
CASTOR. Dose:				
Of the powder,	6 to 8 grains.	3 to 4 grains.	2 or 3 times a day.	} In a little warm
Of the tincture,	30 to 40 drops.	10 to 15 drops.	2 or 3 times a day.	} brandy and water.
Good for convulsions, or fits, and nervous weakness.				
COLCHICUM. Dose:				
Of the wine,	1 teaspoonful.	10 to 15 drops.	2 or 3 times a day.	In a little water.
Of the oxymel,	do.	10 to 15 drops.	2 or 3 times a day.	In a little water.
Good for weakness after illness, coughs, rheumatism, gout, and asthma.				
CARDAMINE, or Lady Smock.				
CINCHONA, or Peruvian Bark. Pale. Red. Pale.				
CONIUM, or Hemlock. Various preparations.				

ANTISPASMODICS.—Continued.

	FOR A GROWN PERSON.	FOR A CHILD FROM 5 TO 7 YEARS OF AGE.	HOW MANY TIMES A DAY.	IN WHAT TO BE TAKEN.
COPPER. Prepar'ns.				
Hippo, or Ipecacuanha	3 to 5 grains.	1 or 2 grains.	Every day.	In warm water.
Hoffman's anodyne,	26 to 30 drops.	6 to 8 drops.	2 or 3 times a day.	In a little water.
Good for hysterics and asthma.				
LOBELIA INFLATA.				
Of the tincture—dose;	30 to 40 drops.	10 to 15 drops.	2 or 3 times a day.	
Of the ethereal tinct'e,	30 to 40 drops.	10 to 15 drops.	2 or 3 times a day.	} In a little water.
Of the oxymel,	2 to 3 teaspoonfuls.	Half a teaspoonful.	Once or twice a day.	
Of the extract,	A half to 1 grain.	Seldom given.	2 or 3 times a day.	Rolled into a pill.
Good for asthma and bad coughs.				
MUSK. Dose:				
Of the powder,	6 to 8 grains.	3 to 4 grains.	2 or 3 times a day.	In a little water.
Of the tincture,	3 to 4 teaspoonfuls.	1 teaspoonful.	Once or twice a day,	In warm water.
Good for convulsions and spasms of the bowels, and nervousness. Also, a stimulant.				
OPIUM—Of the gum or powder,	A half to 1 grain.	One fourth grain.	Once or twice a day.	In a pill, rolled with gum Arabic.
Of the tincture or wine, called laudanum,	15 to 20 drops.	5 to 8 drops.	Once or twice a day.	In water.

The gum or powder good for colics, cramps, and pains of the bowels. The tincture or wine, for restlessness and to relieve pain.

ANTISPASMODICS.—Continued.

	FOR A GROWN PERSON.	FOR A CHILD FROM 5 TO 7 YEARS OF AGE.	HOW MANY TIMES A DAY.	IN WHAT TO BE TAKEN.
PAREGORIC Elixir. Dose:	1 to 2 teaspoonfuls.	10 to 20 drops.	2 or 3 times a day.	In a little water.
Good for weakness of the stomach, asthma, cramps and pains in the bowels.				
PEPPERMINT—Of the essence. Dose:	10 to 20 drops.	8 to 10 drops.	2 or 3 times a day.	On a lump of sugar.
Good for wind in the bowels.				
POPPIES (white). Of the syrup,	3 to 5 teaspoonfuls.	1 teaspoonful.	Once or twice a day.	In a little water.
Good for colics, pains of the bowels, and coughs. Also, good in asthma.				
TOBACCO. Dose: Of the wine,	$\frac{1}{4}$ to 1 teaspoonful.	5 drops.	Once or twice a day.	In water.
Good for asthma, cramps, spasms, and convulsions. Also, in obstinate coughs.				
☞ *This medicine must be used with great care, as it is sometimes very severe in its effects.*				
VALERIAN. Dose: Of the tincture,	50 to 60 drops.	20 to 30 drops.	2 or 3 times a day.	In water.
Of the volatile tinct.,	50 to 60 drops.	20 to 30 drops.	2 or 3 times a day.	In water.
Good for headaches, low spirits, and nervousness. Also, for weakness and giddiness.				

ABSORBENTS, *or such Medicines as are* used *to relieve Acidity of the Stomach and Bowels. An Emetic or Purge should be given, generally, before using them, although they may be given without.*

	FOR A GROWN PERSON.	FOR A CHILD FROM 5 TO 7 YEARS OF AGE.	HOW MANY TIMES A DAY.	IN WHAT TO BE TAKEN.
AMMONIA (Carbonate), or salt of Hartshorn. Dose: ☞ This preparation is not often used, and is not equal to the Aqua Ammonia, or Hartshorn.				
HARTSHORN. Dose:	30 to 40 drops.	6 to 8 drops.	Once or twice a day.	In water.
Good for low spirits, fainting, and nervousness.				
CHALK (crab's eyes), or the prepared. Dose:	8 to 10 grains.	3 to 4 grains.	Once or twice a day.	In little mint-water.
Good for acid stomach and loose bowels.				
LIME-WATER. Dose:	3 to 4 tablespoonfuls	3 to 4 teaspoonfuls.	Once during the day	
Good for acid stomach and heartburn.				
MAGNESIA (Calcined). Dose:	20 to 30 and 40 grs.	8 to 12 grains.	Once or twice a day.	} In common or mint-water.
Of the carbonate,	30 to 40 grains.	10 to 12 grains.	Once or twice a day.	
Good for acid stomach, heartburn, and a gentle purge.				
SUBCARBONATE of POTASH, or prepared Kali, or Salt of Tartar.				
Good for acid stomach, heartburn, and a gentle purge.				

2*

ABSORBENTS.—Continued.

	FOR A GROWN PERSON.	FOR A CHILD FROM 5 TO 7 YEARS OF AGE.	HOW MANY TIMES A DAY.	IN WHAT TO BE TAKEN.
CARBONATE OF POTASH. Dose: Solution of Subcarbonate of Potash, or Ley of Tartar. Dose: Good for acid stomach and heartburn.				
CARBONATE OF SODA.—Subcarbonate of Soda, or prepared Natron:	6 to 8 grains.	3 to 4 grains.	2 or 3 times a day.	In mint-water.
SUPERCARBONATE of SODA:	1 teaspoonful.	4 to 5 grains.	3 or 4 times a day.	In water.
Good for acid and weak stomach, and difficulty of making water, irritability of the stomach and bladder. Also, good in gonorrhœa, or clap.				
BURNT HARTSHORN. Not often used. Good for acid stomach and heartburn.				
BURNT SPONGE, SHELLS (Prepared),				Now and then during the day.
RHUBARB ROOT: Good for acid stomach, and opens the bowels.	Chew a small piece.			

ALTERATIVES, or such Medicines as alter, increase, or improve, the Secretions of the Body, when irregular, obstructed, or bad.

☞ NOTE.—I have taken the liberty of making these a distinct class, to suit the purposes of the work.

	FOR A GROWN PERSON.	FOR A CHILD FROM 5 TO 7 YEARS OF AGE.	HOW MANY TIMES A DAY.	IN WHAT TO BE TAKEN.
ANTIMONY. Of the precipitated Sulphuret or Kermes Mineral,	1 or 2 grains.	One half a grain.	Once or twice a day.	With a little sugar, or in pills.
The Golden Sulphuret,	1 or 2 grains.	One half a grain.	Once or twice a day.	
Good for impure secretions of the skin and blood.				
ÆTHIOPS. Mineral:	10 to 20 grains.	8 to 10 grains.	2 or 3 times a day.	In syrup.
Good for sores on the skin, and scaldhead in children.				
IODINE. Of the tincture—dose:	15 to 20 drops.	5 or 6 drops.	2 or 3 times a day.	In mucilage or tea.
Good for scrofula and enlargement of the glands.				

THE WHITE PRECIPITATE.—Used only, mixed with lard, to destroy vermin in the head.
THE RED PRECIPITATE.—Used to burn and purify foul ulcers on the limbs or body.
MERCURIAL OINTMENT.—Rubbed under the arms, or in the groin, produces salivation. Also, rubbed on to destroy crabs.

THE ACETATE OF MERCURY.—Cures ugly pimples on the face. Take a camel's-hair brush, dip it in, and touch the pimple.

☞ These last four are never given internally.

ALTERATIVES.—Continued.

	FOR A GROWN PERSON.	FOR A CHILD FROM 5 TO 7 YEARS OF AGE.	HOW MANY TIMES A DAY.	IN WHAT TO BE TAKEN.
MERCURY. Of the blue pill. Dose:	5 or 6 grains.	2 or 3 grains.	At night—bedtime.	Rolled into a pill.
Of the chloride or calomel,	3 to 4 grains.	2 or 3 grains.	2 or 3 times a day, or night and morning.	In sugar or pills.
*Bichloride, or corrosive sublimate,	From $\frac{1}{16}$ to $\frac{1}{8}$ of a grain.	Dangerous.	Once a day enough.	In a wineglass of syrup or sugar & water

* This is a poison, and should be handled with great care.
Good for biliousness, costiveness, indigestion, dysentery, when the liver is sluggish, and for venereal diseases, scrofula, and pox, and when in larger quantities, mixed with water, rubbed on to destroy crabs.
☞ The first two preparations are used in several diseases to restore or increase the mucous and salivary secretions, when dried up or checked.

MURIATIC ACID:	15 to 20 drops.	3 to 5 drops.	2 or 3 times a day.	In water, $\frac{1}{2}$ tumbler.

Good for liver complaints, eruptions of the skin, and scrofula.

SARSAPARILLA—(root). Compound decoction. Dose:	1 wineglassful.	1 tablespoonful.	4 or 5 times a day.	In water.
Syrup,	1 wineglassful.	1 tablespoonful.	4 or 5 times a day.	In water.

Good for impurity of the blood, scrofula, and venereal diseases.

BURNT SPONGE:	10 to 15 grains.	5 to 6 grains.	2 or 3 times a day.	In simple-syrup.

Good for scrofula and enlargement of the glands.

ALTERATIVES.—Continued.

	FOR A GROWN PERSON.	FOR A CHILD FROM 5 TO 7 YEARS OF AGE.	HOW MANY TIMES A DAY.	IN WHAT TO BE TAKEN.
SODA—the subcarbonate or prepared natron. Dose:	6 to 8 grains.	3 to 4 grains.	2 or 3 times a day.	In mint-water.
Good for scrofula and sourness of the stomach.				
SULPHUR—the flowers of. Dose:	½ to 1 teaspoonful.	10 to 15 grains.	2 or 3 times a day.	Molasses or honey.
Good for the itch, and eruptions of the skin of a scabby nature. This is also a mild purge.				
MILK of SULPHUR:	Half a teaspoonful.	8 to 10 grains.	Once or twice a day.	In any syrup.
Good for diseases of the skin, sores, &c.				

ANTISEPTICS, *or such Medicines as given internally, or applied externally, prevent a tendency to Putrefactions of the Body, or any parts of it, and are used in such Diseases as malignant Typhus Fever, putrid Sore Throat, and Mortification of the Limbs and Extremities.*

	FOR A GROWN PERSON.	FOR A CHILD FROM 5 TO 7 YEARS OF AGE.	HOW MANY TIMES A DAY.	IN WHAT TO BE TAKEN.
ABSINTHIUM — or common Wormwood, steeped in spirits: Good for weakness after childbirth, and after typhus fever. It may be used, also, after small-pox, varioloid, and such diseases.	A wineglass.	1 tablespoonful.	2 or 3 times a day.	In water or plain.
ACETIC ACID — or distilled Vinegar: Good for foul ulcers about the body and extremities, and for liver complaints. This is an excellent remedy, also, for dropsy, difficulty of passing water, and in clap or gleet.	Half a wineglass.	1 tablespoonful.	2 or 3 times a day.	In water.
CITRIC ACID — of the crystals: Good in putrid sore throat, varioloid, and small-pox. Very pleasant to the patient.	30 to 40 grains.	15 to 20 grains.	3 or 4 times a day.	In water.
CAMPHOR — of the gum: Good for typhus fever and putrid sore throat.	3 to 4 grains.	2 to 3 grains.	2 or 3 times a day.	In powder or pills.
CAMOMILE (flowers). Dose:	Steep a handful of the flowers in a pint of boiling water, let it cool, and give a wineglassful every 3 hours. Good for weakness after illness. Also, a tonic.			

ANTISEPTICS.—Continued.

	FOR A GROWN PERSON.	FOR A CHILD FROM 5 TO 7 YEARS OF AGE.	HOW MANY TIMES A DAY.	IN WHAT TO BE TAKEN.
CINCHONA, or common pale Peruvian Bark.				
Of the powder,	6 to 8 grains.	3 to 4 grains.	3 or 4 times a day.	In hot water, cooled
Of the quill bark, Yellow Peruvian Bark, Red Peruvian Bark,	3 or 4 quills.	1 quill put into boiling water, and allowed to cool.	A wineglassful every 3 or 4 hours.	

Good in mortification from gunshot wounds, and injuries, hospital gangrene, and in all putrefactive diseases. It is also a tonic, and strengthens in weakness from long illness.

LEMON.				
MYRRH—of the tincture,	1 teaspoonful.	Half a teaspoonful.	In a wineglass of water, held in the mouth but not swallowed.	

Good in scurvy and sore mouth.

MURIATIC ACID.				
Dose:	15 to 20 drops.	8 to 10 drops.	Twice a day.	In water.

Good for diseases of the skin, scrofula, and foul ulcers.

NITRIC ACID:	10 to 15 or 20 drops.	6 to 8 or 10 drops.	2 or 3 times a day.	In water.

Good for diseases of the skin, scrofula, and foul ulcers.

☞ Nitric and muriatic acid mixed together, one half a wineglass of each, and thrown into a **bath,** is very strengthening in illness from fevers, &c.

ANTISEPTICS.—Continued.

	FOR A GROWN PER-SON.	FOR A CHILD FROM 5 TO 7 YEARS OF AGE.	HOW MANY TIMES A DAY.	IN WHAT TO BE TAKEN.
OPIUM (in pills): Good for scurvy and foul ulcers.	$\frac{1}{4}$ to 1 grain.	$\frac{1}{4}$ of a grain.	Once or twice a day.	In a pill.
SULPHURIC ACID: Good for diseases of the skin, scrofula, and foul ulcers.	5 to 10 drops.	3 to 6 drops.	2 or 3 times a day.	In water.

☞ Among these, I must mention COLD WATER, applied to the body with a sponge or towel, frequently useful in many of these diseases.

ANTHELMINTICS, or such Medicines as are given to destroy and remove Worms from the Bowels—same as Vermifuges.

	FOR A GROWN PERSON.	FOR A CHILD FROM 5 TO 7 YEARS OF AGE.	HOW MANY TIMES A DAY.	IN WHAT TO BE TAKEN.
ALLIUM, or Garlick.				
ASAFŒTIDA.				
CAMPHOR. Dose:	See page 14 (Antispasmodics) for the dose.			
CALOMEL. Dose:	4 to 5 grains.	2 or 3 grains.	2 or 3 times a day.	In sugar or honey.
Good for all kinds of worms.				
GAMBOGE—of the gum and powder:	3 grains.	1 grain.	Twice a day.	In honey.
Good for worms (generally combined with the same quantity of calomel).				
IRON FILINGS:	8 to 10 or 20 grs.	3 to 4 grains.	Twice a day.	In syrup.
Good for worms, scurvy, rickets, epilepsy, and indigestion. Excellent for the tapeworm.				
JALAP—of the powder. Dose:	8 to 10 grains.	4 to 5 grains.	2 or 3 times a day.	In honey.
Of the tincture,	1 to 2 teaspoonfuls.	1 teaspoonful.	2 or 3 times a day.	In water.
The powder, good for all kinds of worms; the tincture, for worms and disordered stomach; also, a tonic.				
MURIATE of SODA, or common table-salt.				
OLIVE OIL:	1 tablespoonful.	1 teaspoonful.	5 or 6 times a day.	Alone.
Good for worms and costiveness. This is excellent in dyspepsia.				

3

ANTHELMINTICS.—Continued.

	FOR A GROWN PERSON.	FOR A CHILD FROM 5 TO 7 YEARS OF AGE.	HOW MANY TIMES A DAY.	IN WHAT TO BE TAKEN.
SCAMMONY—of the powder:	6 to 8 grains.	3 to 5 grains.	4 times a day.	In syrup.

Good for worms and costiveness. It is generally used with calomel. Mix three or four grains of calomel with each powder. If the scammony is used alone, you must increase the dose.

	FOR A GROWN PERSON.	FOR A CHILD FROM 5 TO 7 YEARS OF AGE.	HOW MANY TIMES A DAY.	IN WHAT TO BE TAKEN.
SPIGELIA, or PINK ROOT:	5 or 6 grains.	3 or 4 grains.	3 or 4 times a day.	In honey or syrup.

Good for worms of all kinds. It is better to give a dose of castor oil and turpentine first. It is better, also, to put three grains of calomel, and three or four grains of rhubarb, in each powder of the pink root for worms.

STEEL.—See Iron.

TANACETUM, or TANSY.—Not often used.

	FOR A GROWN PERSON.	FOR A CHILD FROM 5 TO 7 YEARS OF AGE.	HOW MANY TIMES A DAY.	IN WHAT TO BE TAKEN.
TIN—of the powder:	15 to 20 grains.	8 to 10 grains.	Night and morning.	In honey or syrup.

Good for worms and epileptic fits.

TOBACCO.—Not often used.

☞ There are several kinds of bark used on plantations; but I prefer the castor oil and turpentine, followed by powders of calomel, pink root, and rhubarb, in the proportions directed for worms, further on in the book. (See Worms.)

ASTRINGENTS, or such Medicines as are used to stop or restrain immoderate Discharges from any of the natural outlets of the Body, particularly the Bowels.

	FOR A GROWN PERSON.	FOR A CHILD FROM 5 TO 7 YEARS OF AGE.	HOW MANY TIMES A DAY.	IN WHAT TO BE TAKEN.
ALUM—of the powder:	4 to 8 grains.	2 to 3 grains.	2 or 3 times a day.	In pills or honey.

Good for bloody flux, great looseness of the bowels, and flowing from the womb. This medicine should only be used when the discharge is great and dangerous. Milder astringents ought to be tried first, or small doses of calomel and quinine.

AROMATIC CONFECTION. Dose:	15 to 20 grains.	6 to 8 grains.	2 or 3 times a day.	In water, with 1 or 2 drops of peppermint

Good for cramps in the stomach and bowels, and for purging.

CATECHU—of the tincture:	1 teaspoonful.	8 to 10 or 15 drops.	3 or 4 times a day.	Mint or plain water.

Good for looseness of the bowels, and flooding of long standing. Also, good to check the courses when they are too free.

CHALK, prepared, or Crab's Eyes:	6 to 8 grains.	3 to 4 grains.	3 or 4 times a day.	Mint-water, or water with paregoric.

Good for looseness of the bowels from acid stomach, and for bowel complaints in general. This is good for infants when they are griped. Take three or four grains of the chalk, and rub it in a mortar; then mix it with half a pint of water, and put in twenty drops of paregoric; strain it through a cloth, and give a teaspoonful three or four times a day.

ASTRINGENTS.—Continued.

28

	FOR A GROWN PERSON.	FOR A CHILD FROM 5 TO 7 YEARS OF AGE.	HOW MANY TIMES A DAY.	IN WHAT TO BE TAKEN.
CHALK, powder, with opium:	10 grains.	5 or 6 grains.	3 or 4 times a day.	In mint-water.
Good for dysentery, and bowel complaints of long standing.				
KINO—tincture of the gum:	1 teaspoonful.	15 to 20 drops.	4 or 5 times a day.	In water with sugar.
Good for obstinate looseness of the bowels, and bloody flux.				
LEAD (sugar of lead).	Apply to a physician for the dose.			
OAK & GALL NUTS				
Good for weak and irritable stomach and bowels, diarrhœa, and looseness.				
LOGWOOD—of the decoction:	1 wineglassful.	1 tablespoonful.	3 or 4 times a day.	In water.
Good for looseness of the bowels.				
OPIUM—the different prepar'ons of opium.				
ZINC—the sulphate or white vitriol.				
TONICS (generally).	Most of the tonics are astringents.			

ANODYNES, or such Medicines as are used to relieve Restlessness, Nervousness, Pain, and to produce Sleep and quiet. They are mild Narcotics, and are used frequently, in large doses, as Narcotics.

	FOR A GROWN PERSON.	FOR A CHILD FROM 5 TO 7 YEARS OF AGE.	HOW MANY TIMES A DAY.	IN WHAT TO BE TAKEN.
OPIUM (purified gum)	1/2 to 1 grain, in pill.	1/4 of a grain.	Once or twice a day.	Rolled in the fingers
Of the tincture, or laudanum,	20 to 30 drops.	8 to 10 drops.	Once or twice a day.	In water.

Good to relieve pain, restlessness, to produce sleep, for asthma, hooping-cough, and spasms.

PAREGORIC—elixir,	1 teaspoonful.	20 to 30 drops.	Once or twice a day.	Water or warm tea.

Good for hooping-cough, asthma, weak stomach, cramp, and restlessness.

POPPIES—syrup of the white:	1 to 2 teaspoonfuls.	1 teaspoonful.	2 or 3 times a day.	In water or by itself.

Good for coughs, restlessness, nervous irritation, soreness and weakness of the chest.

TINCTURE of HYOSCIAMUS, or Henbane:	20 to 40 drops.	6 to 8 drops.	3 or 4 times a day.	In sugar and water. It acts also on the kidneys, producing a flow of urine.

Good for shortness of breath, consumption, weakness and soreness of the chest.

TOBACCO—of the wine:	30 to 60 drops.	10 to 15 drops.	2 or 3 times a day.	In water.
Of the extract (not often used):	2 to 3 grains.	1/2 a grain.	Once or twice a day.	In a pill.

Good for bronchitis, violent, spasmodic coughs, cramp and spasmodic closure of the windpipe, asthma.

3*

APERIENTS, or such Medicines as open the Bowels gently—same as mild Purges.

	FOR A GROWN PERSON.	FOR A CHILD FROM 5 TO 7 YEARS OF AGE.	HOW MANY TIMES A DAY.	IN WHAT TO BE TAKEN.
CREAM of TARTAR.	1 to 2 teaspoonfuls.	30 to 40 grains.	Once or twice a day.	In sugar and water.
Good for eruptions and sores of the skin, and erisipelas.				
RHUBARB—root.				
The plain tincture,	2 to 3 teaspoonfuls.	1 teaspoonful.	4 or 5 times a day.	With a little sugar and water.
Compound tincture,	2 to 3 teaspoonfuls.	1 teaspoonful.	4 or 5 times a day.	
Of the wine,	3 to 4 teaspoonfuls.	2 teaspoonfuls.	3 times a day.	In sugar and water.
Good for cramps, wind in the bowels, and stomach-ache.				
SAL POLYCREST:	1 teaspoonful.	½ a teaspoonful.	2 or 3 times a day.	In water, ½ tumbler.
Cooling purge, and keeps the bowels gently open. This mixture is an excellent substitute for the sulphur water of the Virginia springs.				
ROCHELLE SALT:	2 to 3 teaspoonfuls.	1 teaspoonful.	Once or twice a day.	In water.
Opens the bowels; cooling.				
SULPHATE of POTASH, or Vitriolated Tartar:	1 teaspoonful.	½ a teaspoonful.	Once or twice a day.	In water.
Cooling purge. Good for eruptions of the skin.				
TAMARINDS—preserved: Pour a pint of boiling water over a tablespoonful of the tamarinds. Put in a little white sugar. Very pleasant and cooling in fevers,				
Good to assist other medicines; given to open the bowels. small-pox, scarlet fever, and eruptive diseases, as rashes, &c.				

CATHARTICS, or active Purges—such Medicines as purge out the Bowels briskly.

	FOR A GROWN PERSON.	FOR A CHILD FROM 5 TO 7 YEARS OF AGE.	HOW MANY TIMES A DAY.	IN WHAT TO BE TAKEN.
ALOES—of the extract of Spiked,	8 to 10 grains.	3 to 4 grains.	Once or twice a day.	In pills.
Of the powder,	6 to 8 grains.	3 to 4 grains.	2 or 3 times a day.	Pills, or with sugar.
Of the tincture,	1 to 4 teaspoonfuls	2 teaspoonfuls.	3 or 4 times a day.	In sugar and water.
Good for costiveness and worms. Aloes are used, also, with calomel and rhubarb, three to four grains in each powder, given three or four times a day, to force the courses when stopped.				
COMMON ALOES—(Barbadoes Aloes):				
Of the powder,	15 to 20 grains.	6 to 8 grains.	Once or twice a day.	Pills, or with sugar.
Of the extract,	10 to 15 grains.	5 to 6 grains.	Once or twice a day.	In pills.
Good for obstinate costiveness.				
GAMBOGE.				
CALOMEL:	5 to 6 grains.	3 to 4 grains.	Twice a day.	In sugar or syrup.
Good for costiveness, biliousness, and a great many complaints. There is, perhaps, no medicine more generally useful than this.				
CASSIA (pulp).				
COLOCYNTH—powder:	8 to 10 grains.	4 to 5 grains.	Every 3 hours, until it acts freely on the bowels.	In sugar.
Good for costiveness (habitual).				

CATHARTICS.—Continued.

	FOR A GROWN PERSON.	FOR A CHILD FROM 5 TO 7 YEARS OF AGE.	HOW MANY TIMES A DAY.	IN WHAT TO BE TAKEN.
COLOCYNTH, of the compound extract:	8 to 10 grains.	5 or 6 grains.	Once or twice a day.	In pills.
Good for habitual costiveness.				
CREAM of TARTAR	1 to 2 tablespoonfuls	1 to 2 teaspoonfuls	2 or 3 times a day.	In sugar and water.
Cooling purge.				
EPSOM SALTS:	1 to 2 tablespoonfuls or more.	2 to 3 teaspoonfuls.	2 or 3 times a day.	In water.
Cooling purge in hot weather.				
JALAP—powder:	15 to 20 grains.	8 to 10 grains.	Twice a day.	In syrup or honey.
Purge in fevers and costiveness.				
MANNA:	2 or 3 tablespoonfuls	Half the quantity.	Until it operates.	
Good to keep the bowels open.				
MAGNESIA—of the calcined:	2 or 3 teaspoonfuls.	1 teaspoonful.	Every 2 hours, until it purges freely.	In plain or mint-water.
Good for costiveness and acid secretions in the stomach and bowels.				
MAGNESIA (carbonate):	4 to 5 teaspoonfuls.	2 to 3 teaspoonfuls.	2 or 3 times a day.	Mint or plain water.
Good to open the bowels, and to carry off acid secretions from the stomach and bowels.				

MERCURY, or QUICKSILVER.—This is not often used. It passes quickly through the bowels, and is used to force obstructions of the bowels in invagination of a gut, &c.

CATHARTICS.—Continued.

	FOR A GROWN PERSON.	FOR A CHILD FROM 5 TO 7 YEARS OF AGE.	HOW MANY TIMES A DAY.	IN WHAT TO BE TAKEN.
OIL,—CASTOR OIL: Of the pure oil, cold-pressed,	1 wineglassful, moderate size.	2 tablespoonfuls, or less.	Once or twice a day.	With a few drops of brandy or mint-water.
The common Plantation Castor Oil (inferior). Give less, as it is apt to gripe.				
Good for costiveness, indigestion, diarrhœa, dysentery, colic, and cholera morbus. Castor oil ought to be kept in all houses, and on all plantations, and is one of the safest and best purges.				
CROTON OIL:	One drop on the tongue. Very severe. Use with caution.			
POTASH—Nitrate of, or soluble tartar.				
Supertartrate, or Cream of Tartar:	Increase the doses directed under Aperients, page 30.			
RHUBARB—powder:	20 to 30 grains, or less.	10 to 15 grains, or less.	2 or 3 times a day.	In mint-water.
Purge for costiveness when the bowels are weak. Rhubarb, in small doses, acts beneficially on enlarged spleens, and in fever and ague. This is not generally known.				
SCAMMONY, powder	10 to 15 grains, or less.	6 to 8 grains, or less.	3 or 4 times a day.	In mint-water.
Active purge in costiveness.				

CATHARTICS.—Continued.

	FOR A GROWN PER- SON.	FOR A CHILD FROM 5 TO 7 YEARS OF AGE.	HOW MANY TIMES A DAY.	IN WHAT TO BE TAKEN.
SENNA—leaves:	2 or 3 tablespoonfuls	2 to 3 teaspoonfuls.		

Pour boiling water over them—say a pint. Give a cupful every two hours during the day, until it operates freely. Good to open the bowels in colds and fevers.

SULPHATE of SODA, or Glauber Salts:	2 tablespoonfuls, or less.	2 teaspoonfuls.	2 or 3 times a day.	In water.

Purge in costiveness, fevers, &c.

SULPHUR—flowers:	2 or 3 teaspoonfuls.	1 teaspoonful.	2 or 3 times a day.	In water.

Purge in eruptive complaints of the skin, as itch, sores, &c.

SALT WATER.—This is used by sailors at sea; it purges actively. Give it by the tumblerful, in the absence of better medicine.

DIAPHORETICS—or Sweats, or such Medicines as produce Perspiration and Sweating.

	FOR A GROWN PERSON.	FOR A CHILD FROM 5 TO 7 YEARS OF AGE.	HOW MANY TIMES A DAY.	IN WHAT TO BE TAKEN.
ANTIMONY—the oxide, or Antimonial powder:	4 grains.	2 grain.	3 or 4 times a day.	In sugar.
Good in fevers and chest complaints, as pleurisy, pneumonia, &c. This powder may be given either by itself or in warm snake-root tea. It is excellent in small-pox, scarlet fever, and measles.				
ANTIMONIAL WINE	1 teaspoonful or less	20 drops.	3 or 4 times a day.	In water.
Good in fevers and chest complaints; also, in erysipelas, or St. Anthony's fire.				
AMMONIA—Carbonate, or Salt of Hartshorn.				
SOLUTION, or AQUA AMMONIA:	20 drops.	8 to 10 drops.	3 or 4 times a day.	In water.
Good for typhus fever, and other fevers, where there is great debility.				
LIQUOR of the ACETATE of AMMONIA, or Spirit of Mindererus:	1 to 3 teaspoonfuls.	1 teaspoonful.	3 or 4 times a day.	In water.
Good in fevers where there is weakness, pleurisy, typhoid, and pneumonia.				
CAMPHOR—Gum:	3 to 4 grains.	1 to 3 grains.	3 or 4 times a day.	In a julep or pill.
Good in fevers and illness, where there is great weakness.				

DIAPHORETICS.—Continued.

	FOR A GROWN PERSON.	FOR A CHILD FROM 5 TO 7 YEARS OF AGE.	HOW MANY TIMES A DAY.	IN WHAT TO BE TAKEN.
DOVER'S POWDER	5 to 6 grains.	3 to 4 grains.	2 or 3 times a day.	By itself, with sugar, or in warm tea.
Good in pleurisy, pneumonia, colds, and winter fevers.				
GUAIACUM—Gum:	5 to 10 grains.	3 to 4 grains.	2 or 3 times a day.	In a pill.
Good in rheumatism and gout of long standing,				
AMMONIATED tincture of GUAIACUM	1 to 3 teaspoonfuls, or less.	½ to 1 teaspoonful.	2 or 3 times a day.	In syrup.
Good for rheumatism and winter complaints from exposure. This preparation is useful in puerperal fever, or great weakness after childbirth. For sailors and seafaring people, who are exposed, take it at night, and keep your bed.				
IPECACUANHA, or HIPPO—powder:	2 grains.	1 grain.	Every 3 hours.	In warm water, syrup, or sugar.
Good in fevers. If it produces vomiting, make the dose smaller.				
NITRE—NITRATE of POTASH, or SALTPETRE:	6 to 12 grains.	3 to 5 grains.	2 or 3 times a day.	In water.
Good for fevers, difficulty of making water, and in pleurisy and pneumonia.				
SWEET SPIRITS of NITRE:	1 teaspoonful.	30 drops.	3 or 4 times a day.	In water.
Good for fevers, irritation of the bladder from clap, and in colds.				

DIAPHORETICS.—Continued.

	FOR A GROWN PERSON.	FOR A CHILD FROM 5 TO 7 YEARS OF AGE.	HOW MANY TIMES A DAY.	IN WHAT TO BE TAKEN.
MUSTARD WHEY. SENEKA, or LARGE SNAKE-ROOT (decoction).	2 tablespoonfuls of the root.	1 tablespoonful of the root.		Put it in a pint of water, and boil it down to half a pint. Give a wineglassful, hot, every hour.

Good in pleurisy, pneumonia, typhoid pneumonia, and typhus fever; also, in weakness after any of these complaints. It is excellent in coughs, with a grain of tartar emetic in it, and with four grains of camphor, sometimes.

SERPENTARIA, or SMALL SNAKE-ROOT (infusion).				Take a small handful of the root, pour on it, when washed clean, a pint of boiling water, and let it draw like tea. Give a wineglassful of this, hot, every hour.

Good in colds, pleurisy, chest complaints, and check of perspiration.

OXYMEL, or ACETATED HONEY:	2 or 3 teaspoonfuls.	1 teaspoonful.	3 or 4 times a day.	By itself or in water.

Good for colds, sore throats, and influenza.

LIFE-EVERLASTING—herb (dry).				Take a handful, pour on it a pint of boiling water, and draw to a tea. Give a cupful every hour, hot.

Good for colds in the winter. This is an excellent medicine to use on plantations. It grows in the old fields, and is known by almost every old woman. It is needless to mention the botanical name. It is generally known by the name of life-everlasting, or catpaw.

4

DIAPHORETICS.—Continued.

	FOR A GROWN PERSON.	FOR A CHILD FROM 5 TO 7 YEARS OF AGE.	HOW MANY TIMES A DAY.	IN WHAT TO BE TAKEN.
VAPOR, or STEAM BATH.				
WARM WATER.	In a bath, or given to drink.			
SAGE TEA.	Very gentle and pleasant.			
BALM TEA.	Very gentle and pleasant.			
WINE WHEY.	Take 1 wineglass of Madeira or Sherry wine, half a pint of milk, hot, 1 wineglass of hot water; throw the water into the milk, with a little white sugar; then put in the wine, strain it, and drink the whey hot, without the curd. Taken generally in bed.			

DILUENTS, or such Medicines as are given in large quantities in Fevers, Bilious Disorders, Disorders of the Chest from Colds or Consumptions, Diarrhœa and Dysentery, Gravel and Stone in the Bladder, and Difficulty of passing Urine. They are generally given warm.

	FOR A GROWN PERSON.	FOR A CHILD FROM 5 TO 7 YEARS OF AGE.	HOW MANY TIMES A DAY.	IN WHAT TO BE TAKEN.
BARLEY-WATER.				
BALM TEA.				
BEEF TEA.				
CHICKEN WATER.				
COMMON TEA (hyson, weak), or sugar and water.				
GRUEL.				
TOAST-WATER.				
WHEY.				
Good in fevers, &c.				

DEMULCENTS, or such Medicines as are used in the above Complaints, and many others, and to sheathe and protect the Membranes of the Bowels, Bladder, and Urethra, when inflamed and tender, in Fevers and Winter Complaints, when the Bowels are weak, and the Patient wants Nourishment.

	FOR A GROWN PER- SON.	FOR A CHILD FROM 5 TO 7 YEARS OF AGE.	HOW MANY TIMES A DAY.	IN WHAT TO BE TAKEN.
ARROW-ROOT (Bermuda).—Take a teaspoonful, pour on it a very little *cold* water till dissolved, and add one or two lumps white sugar; pour on them one pint boiling water. This may be made thicker by using more arrow-root. Give a little, warm, every now and then.				
GUM ARABIC (best).—Take a teaspoonful of the powder, one teaspoonful of powdered white sugar; pour on them a pint of hot or cold water, and stir it well. Give a little every now and then.				
ALTHEA, or MARSH-MALLOW.—This must be boiled. Ask a physician or apothecary for directions. Give a little, warm, every now and then.				
ALMONDS (sweet). Of the emulsion:	1 wineglassful, small size.	2 to 3 tablespoonfuls	3 or 4 times a day.	
Good for coughs and stoppage of urine.				
OIL OF ALMONDS:	1 teaspoonful or less	30 drops.	3 or 4 times a day.	In syrup.
Good for coughs, clap, and difficulty of making water.				
BARLEY (pearl).—Boil it with a plenty of water.				
CARRAGEEN, or IRISH MOSS.—Prepared same as litchen.				
FLAXSEED.				
LITCHEN, or ICELAND MOSS.—Take a tablespoonful, pour on it a pint of water, boil down to half a pint; sweeten with white sugar.				

DEMULCENTS.—Continued.

FOR A GROWN PER-SON.	FOR A CHILD FROM 5 TO 7 YEARS OF AGE.	HOW MANY TIMES A DAY.	IN WHAT TO BE TAKEN.

MALLOWS.
LIQUORICE (extract).—Dissolve in hot water. Give a tablespoonful every half hour. Good for colds, check of perspiration, and soreness of the chest.

LIVE OIL (Lucca.) | 1 wineglassful. | 2 tablespoonfuls. |Once or twice a day.|Plain or warm wat'r Good for dyspepsia and costiveness. Dyspeptics should use a plenty of good oil with their food.

4*

DIURETICS, or such Medicines as promote and increase the flow of Urine, and force it when checked or stopped. They are used in Dropsy and Strangury; also in Clap, Gravel, and stoppage of the Kidneys from cold.

	FOR A GROWN PER-SON.	FOR A CHILD FROM 5 TO 7 YEARS OF AGE.	HOW MANY TIMES A DAY.	IN WHAT TO BE TAKEN.
COLCHICUM, or Meadow Saffron (extract):	From $\frac{1}{2}$ to 1 grain.	$\frac{1}{4}$ a grain.	2 or 3 times a day.	In pills.
Of the wine or tinct.,	1 teaspoonful.	30 drops.	2 or 3 times a day.	In water.
Good for rheumatism, and painful affections of the body and limbs from cold.				
DIGITALIS, or FOX-GLOVE (powder):	$\frac{1}{2}$ to 1 grain.	$\frac{1}{2}$ a grain.	2 or 3 times a day.	In water.
Of the tincture,	15 to 20 drops.	8 to 10 drops.	3 or 4 times a day.	In syrup.
Good for dropsy of the chest, and general dropsy, and water about the heart, palpitation of the heart, and shortness of breath.				
ELM.				
JUNIPER (berries):	Boil a handful of the berries, and give a wineglass of the fluid every 3 hours.			
	Good for dropsy, clap, and stoppage of the urine.			
LYTTA, or CAN-THARIDES.				
Of the tincture,	5 to 6 drops.	2 to 3 drops.	2 or 3 times a day.	In water.
PINE GUM and TAR.				
Good in clap and gleet.				

DIURETICS.—Continued.

	FOR A GROWN PERSON.	FOR A CHILD FROM 5 TO 7 YEARS OF AGE.	HOW MANY TIMES A DAY.	IN WHAT TO BE TAKEN.
POTASH—Supertartrate of Potash. (Crystals of tartar.) Good for clap, gleet, and acid stomach.	5 to 6 grains.	3 to 4 grains.	2 or 3 times a day.	In water.
CARBONATE of POTASH. SUB-CARBONATE of POTASH, or prepared Kali. Good in stoppage of urine. A mild alkali.	2 to 3 tablespoonfuls or less.	1 tablespoonful, or less.	2 or 3 times a day.	In water.
ACETATE of POTASH, or diuretic salt. Good for dropsy, stoppage of urine, clap, and gleet. To prepare this on a plantation, take pearlash and vinegar, and mix them together slowly, until the effervescence ceases; then use the liquor.	½ to 1 wineglassful, or less.	2 tablespoonfuls, or less.	2 or 3 times a day.	In water.
NITRATE of POTASH, or Saltpetre: Good for fevers, strangury, burning, and difficulty of making water.	10 to 15 grains.	3 to 5 grains.	2 or 3 times a day.	In water.
Liquor of CITRATE of POTASH, or Saline Mixture.				

DIURETICS.—Continued.

	FOR A GROWN PERSON.	FOR A CHILD FROM 5 TO 7 YEARS OF AGE.	HOW MANY TIMES A DAY.	IN WHAT TO BE TAKEN.
SWEET SPIRITS of NITRE:	1 to 2 teaspoonfuls.	1 teaspoonful.	3 or 4 times a day.	In water.
Good in clap, fevers, and difficulty of making water.				
CARBONATE of SODA.	15 to 20 grains.	8 to 10 grains.	2 or 3 times a day.	In water.
SUB-CARBONATE of SODA, or prepared Natron:	6 to 8 grains.	3 to 4 grains.	2 or 3 times a day.	In water.
Good for strangury and fever, where the urine is scanty and red.				
SARSAPARILLA: Drink freely of the decoction. Purifies the blood.				
SENEKA, or LARGE SNAKE-ROOT:	2 tablespoonfuls of the roots.	1 tablespoonful, boiled in a pint of water to half a pint.		
Good for stoppage of urine, clap and gleet, and winter complaints.				
SQUILLS (powder):	1 to 2 grains.	½ a grain.	Twice a day.	In pills.
OXYMEL of Squills:	1 to 2 tablespoonfuls or less.	1 teaspoonful.	2 or 3 times a day.	

Good for coughs, chest complaints, colds, and check of perspiration.

DIURETICS.—Continued.

	FOR A GROWN PERSON.	FOR A CHILD FROM 5 TO 7 YEARS OF AGE.	HOW MANY TIMES A DAY.	IN WHAT TO BE TAKEN.
TURPENTINE—solidified gum. Good for clap, gleet, and scanty urine.	3 or 4 pills.	1 pill.	3 or 4 times a day.	In syrup.
SPIRITS OF TURPENTINE: Good for gravel, gleet, worms, epilepsy, rheumatism, and neuralgia.	30 to 40 drops.	8 to 10 drops.	2 or 3 times a day.	In syrup.

EMETICS, or such Medicines as produce Vomiting or Puking. They also produce Perspiration and act on the Chest, producing spitting, and on the Bowels, producing purging, and relieve Spasms, Coughs, and assist in producing the Courses in Women, when stopped.

	FOR A GROWN PERSON.	FOR A CHILD FROM 5 TO 7 YEARS OF AGE.	HOW MANY TIMES A DAY.	IN WHAT TO BE TAKEN.
ANTIMONY—the antimonial powder in large doses:	8 to 10 grains.	5 to 6 or more grs.	Until they vomit.	Warm flaxseed tea.
ANTIMONIAL WINE	1 teaspoonful.	½ a teaspoonful.	Every half-hour, till it vomits well.	In a little water.

Good in fever and ague, chest complaints, &c.

TARTRATE OF ANTIMONY and POTASH, or TARTAR EMETIC.	1 grain.	½ a grain.	Put into a tumbler of water, and given every now and then until the patient vomits. Sometimes give all at once.	

Good in measles struck in, biliousness, and in fevers to throw off bile.

SULPHATE of COPPER, or BLUE VITRIOL:	1 teaspoonful.	Not often used.	In water, until it vomits.	
HIPPO, or Ipecacuanha	1 teaspoonful.	6 or 8 grs. or more.	In warm water.	Given till it vomits.
Of wine of Hippo:	2 to 4 tablespoonfuls	In warm water—half for a child.		

Good to throw off sour or indigestible food from the stomach, and in dysentery. Hippo is excellent in small-pox, measles, and eruptive diseases, to throw the eruption out on the skin.

EMETICS.—Continued.

	FOR A GROWN PERSON.	FOR A CHILD FROM 5 TO 7 YEARS OF AGE.	HOW MANY TIMES A DAY.	IN WHAT TO BE TAKEN.
TINCT. of LOBELIA, Good for severe asthma.	1 teaspoonful.			In water.
SQUILLS—powder:	2 to 3 grains.	1 grain.	Once or twice a day.	In syrup or warm water.
Of Oxymel of Squills,	3 or 4 tablespoonfuls	1 tablespoonful.	Once or twice a day.	In water.
Syrup of Squills,	do. do. or less.	1 tablespoonful.	Once or twice a day.	do.
Tincture of Squills,	1 teaspoonful.	30 drops.	3 or 4 times a day.	do.
Good for chest complaints, asthma, and bad coughs.				
TOBACCO:	Very severe. Seldom used but in strangulated hernia and severe asthma.			
SULPHATE of ZINC or White Vitriol. Good in sore throat and asthma.	25 to 30 grains.	8 to 10 grains.	Until it vomits.	In warm water.

EMMENAGOGUES, or such Medicines as produce the Monthly Courses in Females, when checked or stopped. They ought not to be used when there are symptoms of inflammation, or a plethora, or fullness of the system. They are good in Chlorosis, or Green-sickness.

	FOR A GROWN PER-SON.	FOR A CHILD FROM 5 TO 7 YEARS OF AGE.	HOW MANY TIMES A DAY.	IN WHAT TO BE TAKEN.
ALOES—different preparations.	*See Cathartics, page* 31, *for dose, &c.*			
	Good for monthly courses, when they are checked, and the patient is weak, pale, and thin.			
ANTISPASMODICS (generally).	*See Antispasmodics, page* 13, *for doses, &c.*			
	Good when the courses are checked, and there is pain and fullness.			
EMETICS.	*See Emetics, page* 46, *for doses, &c.*			
	Good when the courses are checked, and there is pain and fullness.			
GALBANUM.				
HELLEBORE (black)				
MERCURY—different preparations.	*See Calomel, page* 31, *for dose, &c.*			
MYRRH.				
IRON—different preparations.	*See Tonics, for dose, &c.*			
RUBIA, or MADDER powdered root:	30 grains.		2 or 3 times a day.	In water.
	Good for courses when checked with weakness. Not often used.			

EMMENAGOGUES.—Continued.

	FOR A GROWN PER-SON.	FOR A CHILD FROM 5 TO 7 YEARS OF AGE.	HOW MANY TIMES A DAY.	IN WHAT TO BE TAKEN.
SAVINE—dried.				
Leaves powdered:	5 or 6 grains.			In syrup.

BATHING THE FEET up to the knees in warm water, with mustard. Twice a day.

TONICS—generally. | See *Tonics.*

☞ *See directions for stoppage of the monthly courses.*

5

EXPECTORANTS, or such Medicines as are employed in disorders of the Lungs and Chest, to cause spitting up of Mucus or matter from the Windpipe or trachea, and the Tubes which branch into the Lungs.

	FOR A GROWN PER-SON.	FOR A CHILD FROM 5 TO 7 YEARS OF AGE.	HOW MANY TIMES A DAY.	IN WHAT TO BE TAKEN.
GUM AMMONIAC—powder:	8 to 10 grains.	3 to 5 grains.	2 or 3 times a day.	In syrup.
Good for coughs and asthma.				
ASAFŒTIDA—tinc-ture of Asafœtida:	30 drops to a tea-spoonful.	15 to 20 drops.	3 or 4 times a day.	In water.
Good for nervous weakness, fainting, and hooping-cough.				
VOLATILE SPIRIT of ASAFŒTIDA:	20 to 30 drops.	8 to 10 drops.	3 or 4 times a day.	In water.
Gum—in powder,	6 to 8 grains.	4 to 5 grains.	3 times a day.	In pills.
Good for nervous complaints.				
ALLIUM, or GAR-LICK.				
ANTIMONY—differ-ent preparations.	*See Diaphoretics, page 35, for doses, &c.*			
BALSAM of TOLU:	½ to 1 teaspoonful.	½ a teaspoonful.	2 or 3 times a day.	In water.
TINCT'RE of TOLU,	30 to 40 drops.	15 to 20 drops.	Twice a day.	In syrup.
Good for coughs of long standing, and for weakness and soreness of the chest.				
BALSAM COPAIVA.	20 to 30 drops.	6 to 8 drops.	3 or 4 times a day.	On a lump of sugar.
Good for coughs and colds, clap and stoppage of urine.				

EXPECTORANTS.—Continued.

	FOR A GROWN PERSON.	FOR A CHILD FROM 5 TO 7 YEARS OF AGE.	HOW MANY TIMES A DAY.	IN WHAT TO BE TAKEN.
EMETICS—generally.	See Emetics, page 46.			
HIPPO:	In small doses.			
MYRRH. Good for asthma and coughs.				
MERCURY—some preparations of Mercury. Good for consumption in the early stages.	See Alteratives, page 19.			
SQUILLS—different preparations. Good for water on the chest, coughs, and asthma.	See Emetics, page 46, and make the doses smaller.			
SENEKA, or LARGE SNAKE-ROOT. Good in pleurisy and pneumonia.	See Diuretics, page 42.			
TOBACCO. Good in severe asthma.				
SULPHATE of ZINC or White Vitriol. Good for sore throat and asthma.	See Emetics, page 46, for doses, &c.			
VAPOR OF SULPHURIC ÆHER (inhaled).				

EXPECTORANTS.—Continued.

	FOR A GROWN PERSON.	FOR A CHILD FROM 5 TO 7 YEARS OF AGE.	HOW MANY TIMES A DAY.	IN WHAT TO BE TAKEN.
VAPOR of WATER or Steam (inhaled). Good for sore throat and asthma.				
Some of the DEMULCENTS, as Oil of Almonds, Barley, Liquorice, &c. *See Demulcents, page 40.* Good for coughs and soreness of the chest.				
Some of the DIURETICS, as Colchicum, Digitalis, &c. *See Diuretics, page 42.* Good for dropsy of the chest, asthma, and weak lungs.				

NARCOTICS, or such Medicines as relieve Pain and Irritability, and produce Sleep. They are also called Anodynes, although I have used the term Anodynes to signify the milder Narcotics, and in this sense they are commonly used.—(See Anodynes, page 29.)

	FOR A GROWN PERSON.	FOR A CHILD FROM 5 TO 7 YEARS OF AGE.	HOW MANY TIMES A DAY.	IN WHAT TO BE TAKEN.
ACONITE, or MONKSHOOD:				
Of the tincture, Good in rheumatism.	½ to 1 teaspoonful.		Once or twice a day.	In syrup.
BELLADONNA, or Deadly Nightshade.				
BELLADONNA—Extract.	This medicine is used in neuralgia with considerable success, but is sometimes very severe, and should be used with caution.			
CAMPHOR—of the powdered gum.	See Antispasmodics, page 13, for dose, &c.			
Good in painful rheumatism and neuralgia, and in colic pains of the bowels.				
CONIUM, or HEMLOCK:	1 to 2 grains.		Once—at night.	In a pill.
Not often used. Good for scrofula, schirrus, &c.				
DIGITALIS, or FOXGLOVE.	See Diuretics, page 42, for dose, &c.			
Good for rheumatism, palpitation of the heart, and nervous complaints.				

	FOR A GROWN PERSON.	FOR A CHILD FROM 5 TO 7 YEARS OF AGE.	HOW MANY TIMES A DAY.	IN WHAT TO BE TAKEN.
HYOSCYAMUS, or HENBANE.	*See Anodynes, page 29, for dose, &c.*			
Good for consumption of the lungs, violent coughs, and difficulty of passing urine.				
OPIUM—its prepara-tions.	*See Anodynes, page 29.*			
Good to relieve pain, colic, spasms, cholera morbus, and all painful disorders, as rheumatism, gout, &c.				
STRAMONIUM, or THORN-APPLE. Of the extract.	¼ to ½ grain, increased by degrees to 1 grain: given in epilepsy, gout, neural-gia, and obstinate rheumatism.			
POWD'R of BURNT HARTSHORN—with Opium.	5 to 8 grains.	3 to 4 grains.	Once or twice a day.	In syrup.
Good in fevers from colds, &c., and for restlessness.				
POWD'R of CHALK AND OPIUM.	1 to 2 scruples, or less, more often.	20 to 30 grains, or less, more often.	Once a day.	In syrup.
Good in dysentery and purging of the bowels, with straining.				
COMPOUND POW-DER of HIPPO, or Dover's Powder.	8 to 10 grains.	3 to 5 grains.	At a dose.	In syrup.
Good in typhoid pneumonia, rheumatism, &c.				

REFRIGERANTS, or such Medicines as are used to reduce the Heat of the Body, in Fevers and Inflammatory Disorders.

	FOR A GROWN PERSON.	FOR A CHILD FROM 5 TO 7 YEARS OF AGE.	HOW MANY TIMES A DAY.	IN WHAT TO BE TAKEN.
ACETIC ACID, or Distilled Vinegar. Good in fevers, erysipelas, and scarlet fever.	*See Antiseptics, page 22, for dose, &c.*			Divide the doses, and give them oftener. The dose of these medicines should be divided, and given oftener, as they are apt, when used in this way, to become uneasy and injurious to the stomach.
ACETATE of POTASH, or acetated kali. Good in fevers, irritation of the bladder, and eruptive diseases of the skin.	*See Diuretics, page 42, for dose, &c.*			
AMMONIA (Muriate of Ammonia), or SAL AMMONIAC.				
ALUM (Sulphate of Alumina).				
CATHARTICS (generally). Good in fevers and inflammatory complaints.	*See Cathartics, page 31, for dose, &c.*			
LIQUOR of the CITRATE of POTASH or Saline Mixture. Good in fevers and inflammatory complaints.	*See Diuretics, page 42, for dose, &c.*			

REFRIGERANTS.—Continued.

	FOR A GROWN PERSON.	FOR A CHILD FROM 5 TO 7 YEARS OF AGE.	HOW MANY TIMES A DAY.	IN WHAT TO BE TAKEN.
NITRATE of POTASH, or Saltpetre. Good in fevers and inflammatory complaints.	*See Diuretics, page 42, for dose, &c.*			
SUPERTARTRATE of POTASH, or Crystals of Tartar. Good for fevers and inflammatory complaints.	*See Diuretics, page 42, for dose, &c.*			
SPIRITS of NITRIC ÆTHER, or Sweet Spirits of Nitre. Good for fevers and inflammatory complaints.	1 teaspoonful.	30 drops.	3 or 4 times a day.	In water.
DILUTE SOLUT'N of ACETATE OF LEAD, or Goulard Water: Good in irritability of the stomach, with retching, fevers, and inflammatory complaints.	8 to 10 drops.	3 to 4 drops.	4 or 5 times a day.	In water.
SUPERACETATE of LEAD, or Sugar of Lead.—Dangerous.				
SULPHATE of ZINC, or White Vitriol. Good in inflammatory sore throat, &c.	10 grains or less.	3 to 4 grains.	2 or 3 times a day.	In water.

SIALAGOGUES, or such Medicines as increase the Secretion of Saliva. They are sometimes useful in Dyspepsia and sub-acute Inflammation of the Stomach and Bowels, when their Secretions are dried up.

	FOR A GROWN PER-SON.	FOR A CHILD FROM 5 TO 7 YEARS OF AGE.	HOW MANY TIMES A DAY.	IN WHAT TO BE TAKEN.
GINGER.				
MERCURY, or Quick-silver (the principal preparations).	*See Alteratives, page 19, for doses, &c.*			
Good for dyspepsia and costiveness.				
MASTICK—gum.				
NITRIC ACID.	*See Antiseptics, page 23, for dose, &c.*			
PYRETHRUM, or PELLITORY of SPAIN.				
TOBACCO:	*See Anodynes, page 29.*			
Good for asthma and strangulated hernia.				

STIMULANTS, or CORDIALS—*such Medicines as rouse and support the Powers of the System, when weakened by Disease.*

	FOR A GROWN PERSON.	FOR A CHILD FROM 5 TO 7 YEARS OF AGE.	HOW MANY TIMES A DAY.	IN WHAT TO BE TAKEN.
ÆTHER (Sulphuric Æther).	See *Antispasmodics, page* 13, *for dose, &c.*			
Good for fainting, nervous weakness, and low spirits.				
ALCOHOL, and the different Spirits, &c.	Dose according to circumstances.			
Good in mania-a-potu, sinking in typhus fever, &c.				
ALLIUM, or Garlick.				
ANISE-SEED (oil).	30 to 40 drops.	3 to 5 drops.	2 or 3 times a day.	In water.
ARNICA MONTANA, Mountain Ash, or Leopard's Bane.	Not often used as a stimulant.			
ARMORACIA, or Horse-radish.				
Generally given in combination with other medicines. Good for dropsy.				
ASAFŒTIDA.	See *Antispasmodics, page* 13, *for dose, &c.*			
BALSAM OF PERU.	6 to 8 drops.	3 to 5 drops.	3 or 4 times a day.	In syrup or water.
Good in coughs of long standing, weakness of the chest, and asthma.				

STIMULANTS.—Continued.

	FOR A GROWN PERSON.	FOR A CHILD FROM 5 TO 7 YEARS OF AGE.	HOW MANY TIMES A DAY.	IN WHAT TO BE TAKEN.
BALSAM OF TOLU.	6 to 8 drops.	3 to 5 drops.	3 or 4 times a day.	In syrup or water.
Good in coughs of long standing, weakness of the chest, and asthma.				
CAJEPUT (oil).	Not often used as a stimulant.			
CANELLA (Alba).				
Of the powder,	5 to 6 grains.	2 to 3 grains.	3 or 4 times a day.	In water.
Of the tincture,	1 teaspoonful.	30 drops.	3 or 4 times a day.	In water.
Good for indigestion and weakness of the bowels, with wind.				
CAMPHOR.	See Antispasmodics, page 13, for dose, &c.			
Good in typhus fever, pneumonia typhoides, and great debility in illness.				
CARDAMOM (seeds).				
Of the tincture,	1 to 2 teaspoonfuls.	½ to 1 teaspoonful.	3 or 4 times a day.	In water.
Of the compound tincture,	1 to 3 teaspoonfuls.	½ to 1 teaspoonful.	3 or 4 times a day.	In water.
Good in weakness, and swelling of the ankles after illness. Good, also, in cramps, indigestion, and wind in the bowels, and colic pains.				
CAPSICUM, or CAYENNE PEPPER.	20 to 30 grains.	10 to 15 grains.		In hot snake-root tea, or with white sugar powdered.
Good in colds and fevers in the winter-time, from exposure; also, in fever and ague, in the fall of the year. When you use red pepper in fever and ague, you must give it just as the fever is coming on. Give a wineglass of the snake-root tea with it, every half-hour, hot, until the sweat comes out.				

	FOR A GROWN PERSON.	FOR A CHILD FROM 5 TO 7 YEARS OF AGE.	HOW MANY TIMES A DAY.	IN WHAT TO BE TAKEN.
CARRAWAY (seeds). Of the tincture.				
CINNAMON. Of the tincture,	1 to 2 teaspoonfuls.	1 teaspoonful.	2 or 3 times a day.	In syrup and water.
Of the compound tincture,	1 to 2 teaspoonfuls.	1 teaspoonful.	2 or 3 times a day.	In syrup and water.
Good for wind in the bowels, cramps, and colds.				
BALSAM COPAIVA. See *Expectorants, page* 50, *for dose, &c.*				
This is used rather to stimulate the bowels, the bladder, and the kidneys, than the body generally.				
It is given in gleet, weakness of the kidneys, to excite the bladder, and sometimes for tapeworm.				
CORIANDER (seeds). Tincture.				
GALBANUM—Compound plaster.				
GINGER — different preparations.				
GUAIACUM (gum): Of the Ammoniated	3 to 5 grains.	1 to 2 grains.	2 or 3 times a day.	In a pill.
tincture,	½ to 1 teaspoonful.	15 drops.	2 or 3 times a day.	In water.
Good for dyspepsia, rheumatism, and gleet.				

STIMULANTS.—Continued.

	FOR A GROWN PERSON.	FOR A CHILD FROM 5 TO 7 YEARS OF AGE.	HOW MANY TIMES A DAY.	IN WHAT TO BE TAKEN.
MUSTARD. Good for rheumatism and dryness of the skin, in winter colds.	Used on the body in a plaster or poultice.			
MINT—Tincture of **PEPPERMINT.** Good for pain in the stomach, and wind in the bowels.	5 to 6 drops.	3 to 4 drops.	2 or 3 times a day.	In water, or on lump of sugar.
GREEN MINT—or Mint-Water.				
MYRISTICA—or **NUTMEGS**—of the tincture:	½ to 1 teaspoonful.	30 drops.	2 or 3 times a day.	In water.
Good for cramps of the stomach, wind in the bowels, &c. It is also used in large doses of the powder, from 1 to 2 drachms, in epilepsy.				
OPIUM—different preparations. *See Anodynes, page 29, for dose, &c.*				
Good in putrid fevers, and fevers of a congestive nature.				
☞ NOTE.—It may seem strange that Narcotics should be also stimulants, but such is the fact. Frequently, when they act as Narcotics on the brain, they rouse the bowels, and *vice versa.*				
BLACK PEPPER—powder. Good in intermittent fevers and fever and ague.	30 to 40 grains.	8 to 10 grains.	5 or 6 times a day.	In a pill.

STIMULANTS.—Continued.

	FOR A GROWN PERSON.	FOR A CHILD FROM 5 TO 7 YEARS OF AGE.	HOW MANY TIMES A DAY.	IN WHAT TO BE TAKEN.
WHITE PEPPER.				
SERPENTARIA, or Small Snake-root.	*See Diaphoretics, page 36, for dose, &c.*			
SULPHURIC ÆTHER.	20 drops to 1 tea-spoonful.	8 to 10 drops.	3 or 4 times a day.	In water.
BALSAM OF CANADA, or Canada Turpentine.				Rubbed on the skin, in rheumatism.
COMMON TURPENTINE SPIRITS.	8 to 10 drops or more	5 to 6 drops.	3 or 4 times a day.	In sugar.
Good in rheumatism, worms, gleet, and epilepsy.				
VALERIAN (root)— Of the tincture,	1 to 2 teaspoonfuls.	½ to 1 teaspoonful.	3 or 4 times a day.	In water.
Good in headache from indigestion and disordered stomach, low spirits, &c.				
DIFFERENT PREPARATIONS of IRON DIAPHORETICS— in general.				
TONICS—in general.				

STIMULANTS.—Continued.

	FOR A GROWN PERSON.	FOR A CHILD FROM 5 TO 7 YEARS OF AGE.	HOW MANY TIMES A DAY.	IN WHAT TO BE TAKEN.
LINIMENT of AMMONIA.	To be rubbed on the skin.			
LINIMENT of CAMPHOR.	To be rubbed on the skin.			
COMPOUND LINIMENT of CAMPHOR, or OPODELDOC.	To be rubbed on the skin. Good for rheumatism, sprains of long standing, and swelled joints, from cold and exposure.			
TINCT'RE of SOAP.	Rubbed on the skin.			
COMPOUND SOAP LINIMENT.	Rubbed on the skin. Good in rheumatism, erysipelas of long standing, chilblains, &c.			
PLASTER OF ASAFOETIDA.	Put over the stomach, for irritable and weak stomach.			
COMPOU'D PITCH PLASTER.				
PLASTER of SPANISH FLIES, or FLY BLISTER.	Put over the chest, and other parts of the body, to relieve pain and inflammation, as in pneumonia, pleurisy, &c. The fly-blister is used to relieve inflammations of the body or inward parts generally. When used to relieve inflammations of the skin, the blister should be placed near the inflamed place, but not so near as to inflame it more.			

TONICS, or such Medicines as are used to strengthen and give tone to the Body and System, when weakened by Disease. They are generally used when the Patient has recovered from a fit of Illness, and is weak.

	FOR A GROWN PERSON.	FOR A CHILD FROM 5 TO 7 YEARS OF AGE.	HOW MANY TIMES A DAY.	IN WHAT TO BE TAKEN.
MURIATIC ACID.	See Alteratives, page 19, for dose, &c.			
NITRIC ACID.	See Antiseptics, page 22, for dose, &c.			
SULPHURIC ACID.	See Antiseptics, page 22, for dose, &c.			
ABSINTHIUM, or WORMWOOD.	Take a little handful of the green leaves, and pour a pint of boiling water on it; give a wineglassful, after it has drawn (cold), three or four times a day; or pour a pint of good whiskey on the leaves, in a bottle, and a wineglass twice a day. Good in weakness after country fever and confinement, and restores appetite.			
ANTHEMIS, or Camomile Flowers.	Take a small handful of the flowers, put them into a pitcher, and pour a pint of boiling water on them; when cold, give a wineglassful three or four times a day. Good for weakness and want of appetite after sickness.			
ARNICA MONTANA, or Leopard's Bane.				
ARSENIC—different preparations. Fowler's Solution.	½ a teaspoonful.	20 drops.	3 or 4 times a day.	In water.
Good in fever and ague, paralysis, and rheumatism of long standing.				
BISMUTH, or Oxyde of Bismuth.				

TONICS.—Continued.

	FOR A GROWN PERSON.	FOR A CHILD FROM 5 TO 7 YEARS OF AGE.	HOW MANY TIMES A DAY.	IN WHAT TO BE TAKEN.
CASCARILLA BARK.				
Of the powder,	8 to 10 grains.	3 to 5 grains.	3 or 4 times a day.	In syrup.
Of the tincture,	½ to 1 teaspoonful.	20 to 30 drops.	3 or 4 times a day.	In water.
Of the volatile tincture,	½ to 1 teaspoonful.	20 to 30 drops.	3 or 4 times a day.	In water.
Good for weakness of the stomach after fevers; gout and rheumatism, and sour stomach.				
CINCHONA, or PERUVIAN BARK.—				
Different kinds.	*See Antiseptics, page 22, for dose, &c.*			
Good for fever and ague, and weakness after fevers, and illness in general.				
COLUMBO ROOT.—				
Of the powder,	8 to 10 or 20 grains.	3 to 5 grains.	3 or 4 times a day.	In syrup and water.
Of the tincture,	1 to 2 teaspoonfuls.	30 drops.	3 or 4 times a day.	In syrup and water.
Good for weakness of the stomach and bowels, from indigestion and acidity, or from long illness.				
COPPER — (sulphate of copper), BLUE VITRIOL. AMMONIATED COPPER.				
Good for gout, neuralgia, and rheumatism.				

6*

TONICS.—*Continued.*

	FOR A GROWN PERSON.	FOR A CHILD FROM 5 TO 7 YEARS OF AGE.	HOW MANY TIMES A DAY.	IN WHAT TO BE TAKEN.
CUSPARIA, or, ANGUSTURA BARK. Different prepar'ns.				
GENTIAN. — (compound tincture.) Good in want of appetite, and weak stomach.	1 to 2 teaspoonfuls.	30 drops.	2 or 3 times a day.	In wine or water.
HOPS.				
ICELAND MOSS. *See Demulcents, page* 40. Good in illness where nourishment is required.				
MANUBIUM, or horehound (tea.) Take a small handful of the leaves, pour on them a pint of boiling water, sweeten with sugar or molasses. Good in colds, coughs, and hoarseness.				
MYRRH (powder and tincture).				
SULPHATE of QUININE.				
QUASSIA. Of the tincture. Good for weak stomach from indigestion and acidity.	½ to 1 teaspoonful.	30 drops.	3 or 4 times a day.	In syrup and water.
RED PORT WINE.				

TONICS.—*Continued.*

	FOR A GROWN PERSON.	FOR A CHILD FROM 5 TO 7 YEARS OF AGE.	HOW MANY TIMES A DAY.	IN WHAT TO BE TAKEN.
PREPARATIONS of IRON (rust of iron). Good for dyspepsia, weakness of the stomach, and indigestion.	8 to 10 grains.	3 to 4 grains.	2 or 3 times a day.	In syrup.
MURIATED TINCTURE OF IRON. Good in weakness of the kidneys and bladder, worms, rickets, and epilepsy.	10 to 30 drops.	6 to 8 drops.	2 or 3 times a day.	In water.
SULPHATE of ZINC, Or, White Vitriol. Good in fever and ague. White vitriol is not generally used in fever and ague, or as a tonic, but it is recommended by several writers.	15 to 20 grains.	6 to 10 grains.	4 or 5 times a day.	In water.
OXIDE of ZINC, or, Flowers of Zinc.	Not often used, but recommended by writers for fever and ague, and epilepsy.			

DIRECTIONS FOR MAKING

PLASTERS, BLISTERS, POULTICES, OINTMENTS, &c.

How to make a cold Mustard Plaster, or Cataplasm.—Take one spoonful of mustard, three spoonfuls of wheat or corn flour; mix them together with a little vinegar or water, and spread on a cloth. If too strong, mix more flour; put thin muslin over the plaster.

How to make a warm Mustard Poultice.—Take a half-pint of corn meal, boil it, and mix with it a tablespoonful of mustard, put into a thin bag, hot, and lay on the part.

How to make a Mustard Pedilumium, or bath for the feet.—Take two kettlefuls of warm water, put into a tub, and throw in two tablespoonfuls of mustard ; stir round, and bathe the feet.

How to make a Mustard Bath for the body.—Take a bathing tub, put in warm water, say half full, then put in four tablespoonfuls of mustard, and stir round ; then bathe the body. If it is not strong enough, throw in more mustard.

How to make the Nitro-Muriatic Bath.—Take a bathing-tub, half fill it with blood-warm water; then throw in a wine-glass of nitric and one of muriatic acid—put in your hand, and if you feel your fingers tingle, or your skin smart a little, it is strong enough ; if not, throw in more of the acids, stir the water well and bathe.

How to make a warm Anodyne Poultice.—Take a half-pint of cornmeal, boil it, and stir well into it, while warm, a teaspoonful of powdered opium, more, if necessary ; put it into a thin bag, and apply it.

How to make an Opium Plaster.—Take a teaspoonful, or tablespoonful, according to the size of the plaster, of powdered opium, pour on it enough boiling water to make a paste ; then spread it on a rag, and apply it.

How to make a Bread Poultice.—Take the crumb of wheat bread, mash it up with warm water or milk. You may sometimes put in a little piece of soft soap, or Castile soap, and beat it up to make it light.

How to make a Carrot or Turnip Poultice.—Take three or four turnips or carrots—boil them until they are soft, mash them and apply them warm.

How to make a common Corn-flour, or Hominy Poultice.— Take a half-pint of corn-flour, or corn grist, boil it, put in a little milk, or a teaspoonful of sweet oil, or hog's lard, to keep it from getting hard—put it on warm. You may, sometimes, put in the soap as in the bread poultice.—(See *Bread Poultice.*)

How to make a Flaxseed Poultice.—Take a teacupful of flaxseed, put it into a small pot, and pour on it a teacupful of boiling water. Then put the pot on the fire and let it boil up twice, or three times, until it is ropy enough to spread on a cloth. The ground flaxseed is sometimes preferred.

There are several other kinds of plasters, but you must send to an apothecary's shop, if you wish to use them; such as, *strengthening plaster, pitch plaster, compound galbanum plaster, adhesive plaster, or strap, &c.*

Poultices may also be made of any vegetable or herb which will boil and mash soft, provided they do not inflame the place, such as, potatoes, salsify, spinach, cabbage, tansy, Indian potato, hops, camomile, the soft pulp of the artichoke, squashes, &c., &c.

How to put on a Blister (Fly-Blister).—Take the blister-plaster in roll, scrape off some with a knife, and spread on a cloth or piece of brown paper; if it is hard, hold it to the fire. If you wish to do it neatly, take a piece of adhesive plaster (sticking plaster or strap), and spread the blister on the yellow or sticking side, leaving about an inch of the strap all round (not covered by the blister). This prevents the blister from slipping.

How to dress a Blister.—When it is taken off, spread some of the simple ointment on a rag, and cover the place—taking care to cut the bladders as they rise.

How to make Simple Ointment, or Healing Salve, in a hurry.—Take equal quantities of beeswax and sweet oil, and melt them together.

How to make a Clyster or Injection.—Common Clyster.— Take a little common soap (ley soap) and warm water, mix them well together, and put them into the pipe or bladder, draw it up and squirt it out of the pipe, until all the air is out of it; then oil the end of the pipe with sweet oil or hog's lard, and when you put the pipe into the fundament, be careful to push the point up toward the back-bone, if the patient is lying on his belly, but if he is lying on his back, you must push it down, always pushing it toward the back-bone.

*Purgative Clyster.—*Take a small wineglass of castor oil, a half wineglass of turpentine (spirits) a tumbler full of warm flaxseed tea, and two teaspoonfuls of castile-soap, scraped fine; mix them well together.

*Anodyne Clyster.—*Take a wineglassful of sweet oil (olive oil) two teaspoonfuls of laudanum, half pint of warm water; mix well together. This is very slightly anodyne. Another is made with the oil and laudanum, without the water, and a half wineglass of laudanum, instead of two teaspoonfuls.

Also this: two tablespoonfuls tincture of asafœtida, and half-pint warm water.

*Flaxseed Clyster.—*Boil the flaxseed, not too thick—or, only pour boiling water on it, and strain.

A piece of common soap, cut sharp, and pushed backward and forward in the fundament, will frequently answer all the purposes of a clyster in costiveness.

*Starch Clyster.—*Mix the starch and warm water, not too thick, and use.

Rice gruel, rice water, barley water, gum arabic, and many other substances may be used, and, in fact, any warm oil, or slimy fluid. Injections of tobacco, and other plants, and drugs, are used in particular cases, but as these set down are in common use, they will prove generally sufficient, and a physician must direct others, if necessary.

How to make Gargles for sore throat.—Honey Gargle.— Take two tablespoonfuls of honey, throw them into a teapot of boiling water; put the end of the spout in your mouth, and draw the steam into your throat.

*Vinegar Gargle.—*Take a tablespoonful of vinegar, a half teaspoonful of salt, throw them into a half pint of water, and mix.

Port Wine Gargle.—Take a tablespoonful of red port wine, a wineglassful of water.

Peruvian Bark Gargle.—Take two quills of common Peruvian bark, pour on them a half-pint of boiling water; let it cool, and use.

Kreosote Gargle.—Take a wineglassful of water, put in four or five drops of kreosote ; if this is not strong enough, put in more of the kreosote, according to the tender state of the throat.

There are several other gargles.

How to make the Calomel and Opium Pills.—Take twenty-four grains of calomel, three grains of powdered or lump opium ; rub them together well in a mortar with a pinch of powdered gum arabic, then put in three or four drops of brandy or other spirit ; roll the mass in a plate, and cut into twelve equal parts and roll twelve pills in your fingers, using a little liquorice root powder, or magnesia, or rhubarb, to keep the pills from sticking.

Every family ought to keep a box of these pills in their houses, and every planter should keep them on his plantation.

See Cholera-Morbus. Most pills are made in this way.

How to mix a dose of Castor Oil and Laudanum.—Take a wineglassful of castor oil, put in fifteen or twenty drops of laudanum.

How to mix a dose of Calomel and Rhubarb.—Take five grains of calomel, from five to ten grains of rhubarb (best), make into one powder.

How to mix a dose of Calomel and Jalap.—Take five or eight grains of calomel, ten or fifteen grains of Jalap, make into one powder.

How to mix a dose of Calomel and Dover's powder.—Take five grains of calomel, five grains of Dover's powder, make them into one powder.

A dose of Castor Oil and Turpentine.—Take a wineglassful of castor oil, fifteen to twenty or thirty drops of spirits of turpentine.

A dose of blue pill.—Take five or eight grains of blue pill mass, make it into a pill.

These doses are for grown persons, lessen them for children according to their age.

BILIOUS REMITTING, OR COUNTRY FEVER.

THIS is the fever which is so fatal to those who live on the swamps, marshes, and plantations, in the summer and fall of the year. It is common in the low country of South Carolina, Florida, Georgia, Alabama, Louisiana, Mississippi, and many of the middle and western states.

Symptoms.—Slight chills, immediately followed by flushes of heat, which disappear and return every quarter of an hour, or so, the chills becoming shorter, and the heat increasing, until a fever comes on. At the same time, the patient feels weary and sleepy, but also restless and uneasy, and frequently low-spirited. Frequently, too, he has pains in his head, back, and limbs, and when the fever shows itself clearly, these pains increase, especially those of the back and legs. Soon afterward, the whites of his eyes becomes tinged with yellow, his tongue is covered with a brownish fur, he becomes sick at his stomach, and now and then throws up bile. He feels a fulness and weight in his right side, just about the short rib, where the liver is, and in the left side, also, and about the pit of the stomach. He breathes heavily, and seems distressed. He passes very little water, and that is very deeply colored with bile. His pulse is full and quick, but not strong or hard, and in general, his skin is dry and hot.

The patient lies in this state for some hours, when a gentle sweat comes out over the upper parts of his body, and sometimes over his whole body. The fever has now cooled, but it does not leave entirely, and the pulse is still quick, and the skin warmer than natural. This is what is called a remission, but it lasts only from one to two hours, when the fever again rises as high or higher than it was before. After some time, the fever cools again, as it did before, and goes on, rising and cooling, day after day, until it comes to what is called a crisis, and the patient suddenly gets better, or the fever continues, and becomes more obstinate, fixed, and steady.

This is the general course of these fevers, but they are sometimes very severe and fatal, and there is no disease which shows a greater variety of symptoms. There is one thing, also, which must be noticed particularly. There are two forms of the disease; one in which the fever rises about nine or ten o'clock in the morning; the other, in which it rises not until twelve or two o'clock. Again, in the first form, the patient has a good and a bad day, which are very evident and distinct, more so than in the last form. For instance; although the fever rises regularly every day, yet it is much higher, and the patient is much more ill every other day. If his fever is not so high to-day as it was yesterday, and he is better, to-morrow his fever will be as high, or higher, and he as ill, or more ill to-morrow, than he was yesterday.

This, as I have said, is the general course of these fevers, but they are sometimes so severe, that they have scarcely any remission, and the fever seems to keep at its height the whole time. Another thing must be noticed too. The fever does not always come on in the day, but sometimes in the evening, and during the night. When the first attack takes place, look at your watch, and you will find that the fever will be pretty regular to the hour, in its attacks from day to day, though this is not always the case. Notice this also; in very severe attacks, the chills are generally very slight, and last a very little while, and the fever rises rapidly to its height, which is intense. The patient has a tormenting thirst, very severe pains in his loins and legs, great distress and difficulty of breathing, excruciating headache, sick stomach, and a very distressing feeling of fullness and weight in the stomach.

After these symptoms have continued about twenty-four hours, or a day and a night, they disappear almost entirely, and the patient becomes calm and quiet.

This calm, however, is like the calms which occur in a hurricane. It is very short: the fever returns with fury; the whites of the eyes become yellow, the eyes themselves red and watery, a deadly sickness comes on, and the patient is tormented with a constant vomiting, raging thirst, and a distressing feeling of weight in the stomach. After some time, the fever cools, the distressing symptoms abate, and a clammy sweat comes out over the body.

All this while, the bowels are generally costive. The fever rises and cools, and the symptoms, which I have described, are

7

more or less violent, changing with the fever as it rises or cools, and the disease keeps this course until it either comes to a crisis, and the patient suddenly gets better, or dies. This change for the better or worse, generally occurs in the third paroxysm; that is to say, after the fever has made two of these violent attacks, and cooled off, and during the third attack.— But if the disease continues beyond the fifth or sixth attack of the fever, the patient becomes very weak, and sinks, the remissions, or intervals of calmness between the attacks, are not distinct, the patient becomes delirious, that is, gets out of his head, the skin feels either stinging hot when you touch it, or cool and clammy, like that of a dead person. The pulse generally becomes quick and irregular, though sometimes it is natural, or nearly so. When the disease has advanced as far as this, the lips become of a purple color and swollen, the tongue dark brown, or black, clammy, and offensive to the smell, the eyes dry, or red and watery, the urine either very small in quantity, or entirely stopped, or of a dark brown color, and has a bad smell. The passages are either black, bloody, and in great quantity, or reddish and watery. The belly feels soft and as if it was filled with air, in which state it is said to be tympanitic, and sometimes, just before the patient dies, blood will be discharged from his bowels, or nose, or mouth.

When the disease appears in this form, as I have just described, it is said to be malignant, and it will be generally found that the more sudden and violent the attack is at its commencement, the more violent and dangerous will the disease itself be, and the chills occur only before the first paroxysm, or attack, afterward they do not appear. But when the attack is gradual and approaches comparatively slowly, the disease itself will be proportionately slow in its course.

Notice this. Between these two varieties of the disease, which I have just described, there are several others, which only differ in their degree of violence, and the symptoms which they exhibit, being complicated, either at an early or late period of their course, with inflammations of different organs, as the brain, the liver, the bowels and blood-vessels. The symptoms which appear in these varieties are so various and numerous, as frequently to puzzle the most experienced physicians, and this is the reason, perhaps, why we see physicians resorting to such contradictory practice in different cases. You will find, however, that the two most important organs affected and most frequently affected, are the liver, and the alimentary canal, that is, the stomach and bowels, and the symptoms and violence of the disease will depend upon the organ which is affected. For instance, if the stomach and bowels are the organs chiefly affected, there will be a great quantity of unwholesome bile in them, a thick, yellowish layer of mucus, or slime, on the tongue, which, as the disease advances, becomes dry, cracked, and of a dark brown or black color. The patient has a bitter taste in his mouth, loses his appetite, and frequently has a disgust for every kind of food; his urine becomes muddy and yellowish, he feels a great weight about his chest, his belly is tender when you touch it, and filled with wind, and he has great pain in his head, and pains in his loins and knees. The remissions or intervals between the attacks of fever, are distinct; his tongue is fiery red at the tip and edges, and when the brown or black crust scales off, is smooth, shining, and red; his passages are watery and reddish, like the washings of flesh; he can not pass his water, and has a craving for cool and acid drinks; and, lastly, when his disease is in its last stage, he has great difficulty in swallowing.

This which I have just described, is called the Gastro-Enteric form of the disease.

Treatment of the Gastro-Enteric form.—When you have satisfied yourself that your patient has this form of the disease, which I have last described, give him this:—

> 12 grains of Calomel,
> 12 grains of Jalap (powder),

in syrup, at one dose, or divided into two, if he is a grown person—if a child, give half. Or this:—

> 10 grains of Calomel,
> 12 grains of the compound extract of Colocynth,

made into 4 pills, and to be taken at one or two doses; or,

> 10 grains of Calomel, and
> 2 tablespoonfuls of Glauber Salts,

in water, in three hours after the Calomel. Remember, you can give these doses only at the commencement of the disease, and when the patient is not troubled with throwing up.

After the bowels have been well purged out once or twice, you can give this:—

> 12 grains of Calomel,
> 12 grains of James' powder (best English),

made into four powders, one powder to be given every three or four hours ; but if they purge too much, or produce vomiting, stop with them for a while, and give this:—

A wineglassful of Castor Oil,
A wineglassful of Lemon, or any syrup, and
A teaspoonful of Carbonate of Magnesia,

well rubbed up in a mortar. Give a teaspoonful every hour. Remember the patient ought to have two or three passages every twenty-four hours, during the course of the disease.

If the skin is very dry and hot, you may put the patient into a bath of water, just cold enough to be comfortable, or sponge his body with water, and let it dry off. Give the patient, also, cool drinks of Lemon juice, sugar and water, or of Citric acid, in place of the Lemon; or you may use the Lemon acid. Or, you may give him drinks made of hot water poured on sliced apples, with a little sugar, or fresh orange juice, with water, taking care to let him drink a very little at a time, for if he drinks too much at once, he will vomit. If he calls for cold water, let him have it in small quantities at a time ; it will not be improper while he is taking the Calomel, as many people think. A useful drink is, Flaxseed tea, allowed to become cold, with a little Lemon or Orange juice and sugar in it.

Notice this. As soon as the patient is taken with the fever, lose no time, but give him the medicines which I have directed, and if they purge too much, stop them for a while, and give injections to keep the bowels open.—(See *Injections*, page 70.) Remember, also, that in this disease, Calomel is your main dependence, but do not give it so as to produce salivation, unless you find the patient sinking, and the fever runs over the ninth day, then use the Calomel and Opium pills directed in page 71. (See page 71.) Give one of these pills every two or three hours, until the mouth is sore. You will find, however, that if you keep up the use of the Calomel and James' Powder (as directed in pages 75 and 76), they will answer every purpose, unless the patient's stomach becomes too weak and irritable to keep them down; then give the Calomel and Opium pills, or these powders :—

12 grains of Calomel,
12 grains of Dover's Powder,

rubbed together and made into six powders. Give one every two hours, until you see mucus, or slime, on the tongue; then stop and see if you have broken the fever. If not, go on; but if the patient's stomach is now strong enough, go back to the Calomel and James' powder. As a general rule, whenever in these fevers, or any other, you can produce a mucus or slime on the tongue, you have gone far enough with the Calomel. But if the disease is not checked, go on till the mouth is a little sore. As soon as you find that you have broken the fever, begin with the Quinine, in small doses. I do not like the modern practice of giving large doses; they generally leave the stomach in a bad state, although they stop the fever sooner than small ones. This is a good mixture:—

4 grains of Quinine, to half a pint of water, with 2 or 3 drops of Sulphuric Acid, or Elixir of Vitriol. Give a wine-glassful 4 times a day.

When your patient is getting well, be careful not to let him over-eat himself, or eat unwholesome food, as cholera-morbus or indigestion is very apt to be produced, either of which will bring back the fever.

Treatment of the Hepatic form of the disease.—This is the most severe, and is generally attended with great irritability of the stomach, but not always. See pages 73 and 74, for a description of the symptoms. Read from, "notice this, also," to "bowels, or nose, or mouth," in page 74.

When you notice these symptoms or many of them, you may conclude that the patient has the hepatic form of the disease, that is to say that his liver is the chief organ affected, and is engorged with vitiated and dark bile. You must now lose no time, but try to get Calomel to act upon the patient as soon as possible. If his stomach is very irritable, and he can not keep down the medicines which I have recommended in page 75, you must bleed him, only at the commencement of the disease; afterward, bleeding is dangerous. If this does not quiet the stomach, give 10 grains of Calomel at a dose, mixed with half a grain of Opium powder, and give 2 or 3 grains of Dover's powder every hour. You must, at the same time, keep giving the Calomel, if the patient throws it up, as it is of the utmost importance to get the Calomel to act upon the liver, and open the bowels, to carry off the unwholesome stuff which is in there. If the bowels are not opened quickly by the Calomel, give injections until they are.—(See page 70, for *Clysters.*)

Cover the patient's bowels with a warm mustard poultice.

7*

(See page 68.)   Put blisters to the calves of his legs, and if he seems to be getting weak, put a large strong blister over the liver, on the right side, just over the short ribs.   (See page 69, for directions for *Blisters*.)

If his stomach becomes quiet, use the Calomel and James' powder, as directed in pages 75 and 76.   I have found the Calomel and James' powders the best powders in Country fever, of whatever kind it may be.

If you find the patient begin to get worse, and sink, put mustard plasters on every part of the body where you can find room.   Put hot bricks, or bottles of hot water, wrapped in flannel, to the feet, and in fact, around the body, to keep up an artificial heat; and give wine, good Madeira or Port Wine, by the glassful; if you have not wine, give brandy and water, warm and strong, and give one of the Calomel and Opium pills, directed in page 71, every hour, or every half hour, until you find by the slime on the tongue, that the calomel is beginning to take effect.   If this is slow, give between the pills 4 grains of Calomel, with a quarter of a grain of Sulphate of Morphine, or 2 grains of Dover's powder at a dose.   Again, if you find that the patient's bowels begin to purge very violently, which is often the case in these fevers, give 4 grains of Dover's powder at a dose, and if this does not stop them quickly, use this mixture:—

A tablespoonful of the Tincture of Kino,
A tablespoonful of Paregoric,
30 grains of Crab's eyes, or prepared chalk,

well mixed up and shaken together with a half-pint of water. Give a tablespoonful of this every half hour, until they are checked, then stop.   While you are giving this, keep on with the Calomel in doses of 4 grains, every hour or half hour.— Don't quit your patient because he seems to be dying.   I have had cases to sink until I could scarcely feel the pulse for several hours, and they could scarcely swallow, and yet they recovered.   Last of all do not let your patient die for want of Calomel.   There are many persons who will not use Calomel, because, they say, that so many people have been killed by it; and I am aware that ignorant physicians have salivated very often when there was no occasion ; but we must not condemn the tools because the carpenter does not know how to use them.   When your patient begins to get better, use the Quinine, as I have directed.

INTERMITTING FEVER, OR FEVER AND AGUE.

A FEVER and ague may be known by the following symptoms ; *the cold stage, the hot stage, and the sweating stage.*

The Cold Stage.—Before describing the cold stage, I will give the symptoms which show themselves, just before it comes on. A feeling of great weariness, a desire to yawn and stretch frequently, slight pains in the loins and legs, and sometimes pain in the back, and melancholy feelings. After these feelings have lasted for some time, the patient begins to feel cold along his back, as if cold air was blowing on him; his fingers and feet become cold, and sometimes shrivelled and pale, and the finger-nails look blue ; he feels restless and uneasy, and is generally cross and fretful, or dull and gloomy. This feeling of cold on the back, soon extends until the whole body has the same feeling to the patient. His skin becomes pale, shrivelled, and rough, his pulse becomes small, but quick and hard, and at the same time weak. And now a shivering and trembling of his jaws come on, which soon extend to his whole frame. The rigors are now said to have come on, and they are sometimes so severe, that the patient seems to be in convulsions. Several other symptoms now make their appearance, which vary according to the age and constitution of the patient, but it is not important to mention them.

After these chills and rigors have lasted some little time, flushes of heat pass over the body and face, which soon increase, while the chills disappear, and the body soon becomes hot. This is the hot stage.

The Hot Stage.—As soon as this stage comes on, the countenance becomes flushed and full, the skin hot and dry, the mouth dry, and the patient has a great thirst. His pulse is strong, full, and quick ; his breathing is more free and regular than in the cold stage, but still more hurried than natural. He has frequently pain in his forehead, and in his back, and legs, and sometimes he is out of his head. The hot stage is generally much longer than the cold stage, but the length of time which it lasts, is different in different cases. After this stage comes the

Sweating Stage.—As soon as the sweat comes out about the head and the breast, the fever begins to cool, the pulse falls, but is still full; the breathing becomes free and natural, and as soon as the sweat comes out all over the body, the fever leaves entirely, but the patient feels languid and weary, and has no appetite, and can not bear cold air to blow on him;—sometimes the patient feels very well, but not often.

This which I have described, is an Intermittent Fever, as it usually occurs; but they are very various in their symptoms, appearances, and character in general, according to the age and constitution of the patient whom they attack.

We frequently see them of an inflammatory character (that is, showing inflammation of some organs of the body), sometimes of a congestive character (or where the blood is disposed to become stagnant in the blood-vessels). Sometimes they appear of a bilious character, and show symptoms of irritation of the stomach and bowels, and sometimes of a malignant character, though not often.

Again. They are of various types, as we say; for instance, when the fever comes on every day (that is every 24 hours), at a regular hour, we call it a regular quotidian fever; when it comes on every other day, at a regular hour, we call it a regular tertian; when it comes on every fourth day, we call it a quartan; and, when it comes on every fifth day, a quintan. When the fever does not come on at the same hour, or near it, we say it is irregular. I shall describe, first, the treatment of Fever and Ague, as it usually appears.

Treatment.—When you see that the disease is a simple and regular or irregular Fever and Ague, as I have described, examine the patient's tongue; if it is foul, and he is sick at his stomach, vomits bile, has a bitter taste in his mouth, pain in his stomach and bowels, or some of these symptoms, you may be sure that his stomach and bowels have unwholesome stuff in them, which ought to be brought away.

Give him one or two grains of Tartar emetic in a tumbler of water, just before the cold stage comes on, until he vomits freely. As soon as his stomach is settled, give him eight or ten grains of Calomel, and when this has purged him freely, begin with the Calomel and James' Powder, as directed in pages 75 and 76. Follow the directions in page 75, also.

While the patient has the fever on him, let him drink freely of cool, acidulated drinks, as lemon juice, or any of the drinks described in page 76, in small draughts at a time, and during the intermission, or while the patient seems to be comparatively well, this mixture I have found excellent.

Take a little handful of small Snake Root, pour a pint of boiling water on it in a teapot; then put in

 12 grains of Dover's Powders,
 1 teaspoonful of Saltpetre,
 1 teaspoonful of Epsom or Glauber Salts,
 1 teaspoonful of Spirits of Nitre,
 1 teaspoonful of Paregoric,
 1 teaspoonful of Antimonial Wine.

Keep this warm by the fire, and give a wineglassful every hour, during the intermission. If the stomach becomes irritable, you must give a Calomel and Opium pill every 3 hours, until it is settled.—(See page 71.)

In this fever, as in Remitting fever, you will find Calomel the best medicine which you can use, only give it in smaller doses. When you succeed in breaking the fever, give the Quinine, as directed in page 77. Remember, also, what I have said about the tongue being slimy. When this takes place, the fever generally leaves or decreases.

In cases where there are symptoms of inflammation, with a strong, full pulse, bleeding is good, and I like bleeding in the cold stage. A few ounces of blood will generally be sufficient. In these cases you will have to use your own judgment and notice the symptoms. As a general rule, although warm drinks are good before the cold stage comes on, never give stimulating drinks unless the patient is very weak, and the cold stage lasts a long time. The stimulating drinks increase the fever when it comes on.

When the patient is getting better, let him change the air if he can, and notice the directions in page 77. With regard to the other forms of the disease, which I have mentioned, I will only say, use your judgment and follow this general rule.

RULE.—Purge out the bowels regularly, but mildly, until all the vitiated stuff comes away, and use Calomel and James' powder, or the other combinations which I have set down, regularly, but with proper caution, until you see the tongue look good, the passages have a yellow and healthy look, and the fever breaks. As long as the tongue is dry and harsh, and

the passages are dark or clay-colored, or ash-colored, keep
on giving the Calomel.

The patient should have one or two good passages a day,
and you should examine them. When you find the Calomel
gripes, stop it for a while, and use the mixture of Castor Oil
and Magnesia, in page 76. You must also increase the quantity of Quinine every day, giving one fourth more.

YELLOW FEVER.

Symptoms.—A feeling of sudden giddiness at the commencement of the disease, weakness, pain in the back, loins,
and legs, sickness at the stomach, and chills creeping all over
the body. After some time, say from 6 to 12 hours, the pulse
rises and beats violently, the skin becomes very hot and dry,
the eyes red, the face flushed; the patient has great thirst,
severe headache, pains in the small of the back and legs, feels
a great weight and tightness about the stomach, and can not
bear the light. His tongue looks white and sometimes clean,
and in about twenty-four hours from the time he was taken,
the patient begins to throw up often, particularly after drinking anything. At first he throws up only such fluids as he
has drank, but after these have come away, he brings up a
quantity of bile, either of a pale yellow or dark green color,
and this is frequently so acid as to make the throat and lips
sore. And now he feels great heat and tenderness about the
pit of the stomach, he looks very much distressed, and quite
hopeless; he sighs frequently, and is very restless, and frequently is delirious. Sometimes he has a difficulty of swallowing, and he suffers from hunger, while he is unable to
move his legs.

This paroxysm lasts, that is to say, the patient lies in this
state from 24 to 36 hours, and sometimes longer, when all the
distressing symptoms, except the sickness at the stomach and
throwing up, are relieved; the pulse becomes natural and the
skin becomes cool and moist. The patient, sometimes, now
seems so much better, that he is inclined to think that he has
got over the attack; but more frequently he seems to be in a
state of stupor, and notices or cares about nothing. This calm,

hewever, like that mentioned in remittent fever (page 73), is ominous; for after a few hours, the pain and burning in the stomach increase and become very distressing; he throws up often and very violently; the stuff which comes from his stomach now has no bile in it, but looks like the grounds of Port wine in a fluid. His thirst is great, but everything which he swallows is thrown up immediately, with great violence. His eyes and the skin about his neck and breast now become yellow.

This second paroxysm lasts, that is to say, the patient lies in this second state just described, from 12 to 36 hours, when new symptoms make their appearance, and the third and last stage of the disease comes on.

His pulse now becomes very weak, his tongue dark brown or black; he throws up every moment, and with violence, and the stuff which comes up, is a black, ropy fluid, like coffee grounds mixed with a glairy, shining fluid. His hands and feet become cold and clammy, and the pain and burning at the pit of the stomach are excruciating. At this time, too, he generally has green or black passages, and feels unable to pass his stools from weakness of the muscles of the belly. And now the whole body is of a dirty yellow color, and the patient soon dies with hiccough, bleeding from different parts, delirium, stupor, or convulsions.

This is the usual course of this disease, but it is frequently much more severe, and, as in many other diseases, has various other symptoms, and assumes various degrees of violence. Sometimes the patient becomes raving mad, or falls down suddenly, as if struck with a blow, and goes off into convulsions, and sometimes the patient sinks and dies before any one thinks that anything is the matter with him, his only symptoms being melancholy looks, and a great change in his temper.

Treatment.—Bleed at the commencement of the disease, but only at the commencement. Take blood until the patient seems fainty. The blood ought to be drawn during the first twelve hours. Give, also,

10 grains of Calomel,
10 grains of Jalap,

at a dose, in syrup, if the patient is a grown person; if a child, less. As soon as the medicine begins to operate on the bowels, help it, by giving injections. (See *Injections*, page 70.) And when the bowels are well emptied, begin with the Calomel regularly; give four grains every three hours, and if you find the stomach too weak to keep it down, stop it and give a Calomel and Opium pill every hour. (See page 71.) Go on using the Calomel at your discretion, until you find that it has had a decided mercurial effect upon the system, then stop and give injections. The bowels must be kept well open during the whole course of the disease.

If you find the pulse very high and symptoms of inflammation still going on, bleed cautiously from time to time, and use fomentations of flannel wrung out in hot water, over the pit of the stomach; you may also apply leeches in this place. When you have subdued the inflammation in this way, use the Calomel as I have directed, steadily, and look frequently at your patient's tongue and passages. If, however, you find at the commencement of the disease, that the patient seems very nervous and oppressed, impatient and irritable, or if as in a state of intoxication, and sinking down careless and desponding, with no signs of inflammation, and a low pulse, you must not bleed, but lose no time in salivating. For this purpose take

12 grains of blue pill,

12 grains of the compound Extract of Colocynth,

2 grains of Sulphate of Morphine,

make them into four pills, and give one pill every two hours, until they salivate. Or, use this;

12 grains of Calomel,

3 grains of Sulphate of Morphine;

made into six powders, one to be given every two hours. Or, give two of the Calomel and Opium pills every two hours. (See page 71.) If, after all this, the patient seems to be sinking, follow the directions for Remitting fever, last stage. (See page 78.)

TYPHUS FEVER.

Symptoms.—An uneasy feeling in the pit of the stomach, loss of appetite, a pale, shrivelled, and dejected countenance, giddiness in the head, and sickness at the stomach; the eyes dull and heavy, a trembling of the hands, a disinclination to move about, and a feeling of weakness and weariness over the whole body. The patient remains in this state from three to six days, when slight chills, followed by flushes of heat, are felt every now and then. The patient feels sick at his stomach and has a disgust for every kind of food; his tongue is covered with a thin whitish fur; he sometimes throws up, and his pulse is quick, small, and irregular. He has, also, a confused and heavy feeling in his head, and he becomes more and more depressed in mind and body.

He lies in this state from six to twelve hours, when the fever comes on. Notice this: his skin becomes dry, his face slightly flushed, his pulse becomes stronger and fuller, he has a thirst for cool drinks, his tongue becomes more furred and slimy, his bowels are costive, he is a little wandering and confused, restless, and fretful; his countenance has a watchful and anxious expression, his urine is reddish and small in quantity; his head feels heavy and giddy, and occasionally, during the nights of the first two days after this stage comes on, he is delirious.

About the end of the second and during the third day of this stage, his eyes become watery, and the blood-vessels in them seem red and full, his throat is a little sore and painful in swallowing; there is a weight about his chest, and he generally has a short dry cough. He has frequently, also, a fullness and tenderness in his right side about the short ribs, pains in his back, loins and legs, and frequently a soreness over his whole body.

Toward the end of the third day, after the symptoms which I have just described, have appeared, he feels much giddiness and heaviness in his head, as if he had taken Opium, or some narcotic; his hearing now becomes dull; he becomes more and more delirious, and a general dullness and stupor comes over him, and in some cases, the skin, at this time, becomes rough, like what is called goose-flesh.

One of the surest symptoms of Typhus fever, is from the commencement of the attack, to the end, a great dislike in the patient to move and exert himself, or to interest himself about anything around him. He gives you short, peevish answers, and seems inclined to be in one position.

The stage of excitement, or fever, which I have just described, usually lasts about six or seven days, and ends in the *Collapse, or Sinking Stage.* Some times it lasts a longer or shorter time, according to the age of the patient, &c. The

collapse may be known by the decrease of the symptoms described in the stage of excitement, great weakness, the pulse
becoming quicker and weaker, the tongue becoming dry,
brown, and at last black, the teeth and inside of the lips covered with a black crust, the patient appearing as if confused
or stunned, and frequently out of his mind, and muttering,
picking at the bed clothes, the muscles of his face twitching,
a great difficulty in putting out his tongue, lying constantly
on his back, and sliding down by degrees to the bottom of
the bed; a stinging heat of his skin, a deep, hollow voice, and
in very violent cases, dark spots on his skin, hiccough, and a
puffy state of his belly.

During the collapse, the urine generally comes away plentifully, and frequently foams like beer; the bowels are generally loose, too, about the end of this stage, and the passages are watery, very offensive, and make the fundament
sore; and, when the patient is beyond recovery, there is
coma, or a dull, heavy sleep, from which he rouses every
now and then, and sinks again.

The stage of collapse generally lasts from seven to nine
days, when the patient either gets better slowly, or dies. If
the patient is about to recover, you will see a gentle perspiration over the whole body. The heat of the skin will cool
off, the tongue will become moist and clear off along the
edges; the urine will come away more freely, and deposite a
sediment; the patient's brain will become settled, and he will
get a little sleep at times, and sometimes the bowels will
become a little loose. These favorable symptoms, however,
sometimes, do not show themselves until the seventeenth, or
twenty-first day; but generally they occur about the thirteenth
or fourteenth day of the disease. The patient gets better very
slowly, and the weakness of both mind and body lasts for
some time after the fever has left.

These are the usual symptoms of Typhus fever, and if the
disease appears with any other symptoms, they will not be
such as to mislead you, as you will see enough of the symptoms
which I have described, to enable you to detect the disease.

Treatment.—At the commencement of the disease, take
from a half to a pint of blood (if a grown person). An hour
or two after, give an emetic of Hippo. (See Emetics, page
46, table of medicines, for dose.) When the stomach becomes
settled, give 10 grains of Calomel and 10 grains of Jalap, at

one dose, or in two. When the bowels have been well opened, give a powder made of 2 grains of Calomel and 1 grain of Dover's powder, every three hours, until you find the patient's gums tender, then stop and give a small dose of Castor Oil. (See *Cathartics*, page 31, for *dose*, &c.) Or give this:—

12 grains of Calomel,
6 grains of Hippo,

made into 6 powders, one powder to be given every three hours, until the gums are tender, or the disease abates. Let the patient drink freely of warm teas, made of Elder blossoms, or Flaxseed, with a little Spirits of Nitre in them.

General Rule to be followed in treating a case of Typhus Fever.—Keep the bowels gently open, give warm mucilaginous drinks, and as soon as you can get Mercury to act upon the system gently, without purging the bowels too much, or irritating them. When the Mercury purges too much, put small doses of 1 or 2 grains of Dover's powder, with the same quantity of Calomel, and give it regularly. When the patient begins to sink, lose no time, but salivate him gently, as soon as you can. See page 75, Bilious Remitting Fever; use the Mercury in the same way.

In the collapse stage of the disease, many writers recommend Musk and Camphor, and some, an infusion of the Mountain Ash. You can try these if your patient is very ill.

Take one ounce of the leaves of Mountain Ash, pour on a pint of boiling water. Give a wineglassful every hour.

Lastly: if the patient throws up during the first and second days of the disease, and his head is relieved, and his bowels loose at an early period of the disease, they are good symptoms, particularly if he bleeds from his nose about the sixth or seventh day of the stage of excitement. Again, when his stomach is not very painful or tender when you press it, and his thirst is not very great during the stage of collapse, but if he has no desire at all to drink, then it is bad. A moist tongue, also, at this time, and a free and soft, but not quick, pulse, are good signs.

The bad signs are, a change in the expression of the countenance at the commencement of the disease, want of thirst and delirium during the stage of excitement. But when the patient becomes blind, sheds tears involuntarily, swallows with difficulty, can not move his tongue, mutters continually, has a small irregular pulse, distortion of the muscles of the face, pain and tenderness about the belly, sees strange objects, moves his hands continually; picks at the bed-clothes, has loose bowels, passages coming away involuntarily, and an apthous appearance of the mouth, he generally dies, though sometimes recovers.

SCARLET FEVER.

There is, perhaps, no disease which appears under so many grades of violence, from the simplest to the most severe and malignant, as this. I will confine my remarks, however, to the simple form, as a physician must be employed for the severe forms.

Symptoms.—The patient, after having the ordinary premonitory symptoms of fevers in general, from one to three or four days, is seized with slight chills, succeeded by flushes of heat, low spirits, sick stomach, pains in the loins, legs, and head. His pulse is frequent and quick, and his skin hot and dry. Within the first forty-eight hours after the fever comes on, a scarlet eruption comes out, first on the face, then on the neck, body, and limbs, and finally may be seen over the surface of the mouth, throat, and nostrils, and sometimes on the whites of the eyes. This rash gives to the skin the appearance of the shell of a boiled crab or lobster.

At the commencement, or soon after the commencement of the fever, there is a slight soreness of the throat, and some difficulty in swallowing. The face is generally a little swelled, the tongue covered with a thick white fur, through which you may see little scarlet points, its edges and tip are generally red. The skin becomes very hot, and the pulse frequent, quick, and sometimes strong; there is seldom much thirst, and little appetite, much restlessness, sometimes slight delirium during the evening, which generally disappears near morning.

The fever and eruption are generally fully developed on the fourth day, and begin to decline on the fifth, and disappear entirely about the end of the seventh day. On the eighth day, the skins begins to scale off.

Treatment.—When you have satisfied yourself that the patient has scarlet fever, give one or two doses of castor oil, or

Cream of Tartar, until the bowels are well opened; gargle the throat (if sore) with sage tea, with a little honey in it, and a small piece of Alum. If the patient's pulse is high, take a little blood, and if he complains of a weight at his stomach, give an emetic of Hippo. (See *Emetics*, page 46, for dose.) Give, also, cooling and acidulated drinks as lemonade, and give as nourishment, a little chicken water or gruel. If the disease does not yield to this treatment, send for a physician.

_____

SIMPLE INFLAMMATORY FEVER.

Symptoms.—Great febrile excitement, great irritability, and power of action in the heart and arteries. The premonitory stage is always short, and the fever comes on suddenly, with distinct chills or rigors, the surface of the body becomes quickly very hot, the pulse full and vigorous, but not often above 112 in a minute; the face is flushed and swollen, the eyes suffused, sparkling, and can not bear the light: the temples and large arteries of the neck throb; the head is painful, the mouth and throat very dry, the patient breathes hurriedly, and with difficulty ; his thirst for cold water is great, his tongue is covered with a white fur, the bowels costive, the urine highly colored and scanty, the skin dry, harsh, and a slight blush may be seen on its surface ; the ears, also, are very sensitive to noise. Delirium does not often occur, but when it does, it is generally very violent, and is a very unfavorable symptom.

These symptoms usually undergo changes, increasing in the evening, and abating in the morning, until a critical day, which is sometimes the seventh, and sometimes the ninth day. When the disease terminates on the seventh day, the symptoms go on increasing in violence to the fourth or fifth day, when they abate. But if the disease is prolonged, the ninth, and sometimes the eleventh day, is the critical day, and the disease, in this case, terminates on the fourteenth day. When the disease is subsiding, a general and free perspiration usually comes out, and you will see a reddish, or pale sediment in the urine. Sometimes the patient bleeds from the nose. All of these discharges usually occur a few hours after the fever has risen in

8*

the evening. These are the usual symptoms attendant on this form of fever, but sometimes other, and very dangerous symptoms occur. You must then send immediately for a physician.

Treatment.—As a general rule, take blood with caution and judgment, to relieve the oppression of the heart; and this must be done at an early period of the disease. You may, however, bleed at any time, if the pulse indicates it. A hard or quick and corded pulse, always indicates bleeding. Next, open the bowels well. For this purpose, use the following;

> 2 large tablespoonfuls of Glauber or Epsom Salts,
> 1 grain Tartar Emetic,
> ½ pint of water,

Give a wineglassful of this solution every hour, until it purges well.

But if at the commencement of the fever, you see symptoms of much bile, give six or eight grains of calomel, a few hours before you give the mixture. After the bowels have been well purged out in this manner, if you find that the brain is becoming affected, give at one dose, 20 grains of Jalap, with 2 teaspoonfuls of cream of tartar, rubbed together with a little honey or syrup. It will be necessary to keep the bowels open during the whole course of the disease (that is, after the remedies recommended above have been administered); for this purpose, give a little cream of tartar (say two teaspoonfuls every day, or twice a day if necessary), dissolved in tamarind water, or the Seidlitz powders. You must be careful, however, not to use purgatives *too freely*, as they may irritate the bowels and do harm.

Diaphoretics, also, will be found useful in this disease, and the best are Saltpetre and Tartar Emetic given together in this manner.

> 1 teaspoonful of Saltpetre (powdered),
> 1 grain of Tartar Emetic,
> 1 teaspoonful of Gum Arabic,

dissolved in a wineglass of boiling water. Add 4 wineglasses of water, and give a tablespoonful every hour or two. If, however, this acts too powerfully on the bowels, stop it and give the following;

> 7 grains of Hippo,
> 1 grain of Calomel;

rub them together and make them into eight powders, and give one powder every hour, or half hour during the day.

Lastly : throughout the whole course of the disease give warm drinks, as flaxseed or balm tea, lemonade or tamarind water ; and use as nourishment (when necessary) chicken water or gruel, taking care to give a little at a time. When the skin remains obstinately harsh and dry, you may use the following powders : —

> 10 grains saltpetre (powdered),
> ½ grain James's powder (English).

Give one of these powders every two hours, until the skin is moist.

COMMON CONTINUED FEVER,

OR SUCH AS ARISES FROM COLD, OR DISORDER OF THE BOWELS AND BILIARY ORGANS.

In this fever, although the excitement of the heart and arteries may at first be as great as in simple inflammatory fever, yet the disease has a tendency to become, very soon, typhoid ; that is to say, the powers of life seem to decrease, and the disease verges to a low state.

It may be known by the following general *symptoms :* When the disease is of a mild form, it comes on with a slight feeling of chilliness, which is soon succeeded by an increase of the heat of the skin (not very great, however). The tongue becomes white, the pulse becomes somewhat more frequent, quick, and full; there is a languor of mind and body, some pain over the eyebrows, a dry skin, urine red and somewhat smaller in quantity. The sleep is disturbed, and the bowels costive, or slow. When the disease appears in this form, it is not dangerous, and generally passes off in a few days (with suitable treatment), with a slight perspiration, or looseness of the bowels. But when the disease is ushered in by a distinct cold stage, when there is great lassitude, restlessness, confusion of the brain, difficult and anxious breathing, a weak and quick pulse, clammy tongue, wind in the bowels, sick stomach, or puking, it is of a very dangerous form. ·

You will find that the skin soon becomes hot, dry, and suffused with a slight redness. The pulse rises and becomes more frequent; the face becomes flushed; there is a dull, heavy, or throbbing pain in the head; the patient becomes restless, surly, or fretful, and his eyes as well as his mind seem to wander about. His tongue becomes at first white, dry, and harsh, and as the disease advances, dark brown; his urine is generally red, though sometimes pale, and has no sediment. His bowels are bound, and when the passages come away, they are soft and often of a clay color.

From the commencement of the disease, the patient dislikes the light and all noise, and the arteries of his neck and temples usually beat strongly.

These symptoms last for five or six days, without any changes of importance, except that the fever is higher in the morning and during the night. During the nights also of the first four or five days, the patient is rather light-headed, and this last symptom increases until the eighth or ninth day, when he gets better, or falls into a collapse, and remains in a constant state of stupor, picking at the bed-clothes, and sinking from day to day, until about the fifteenth or seventeenth day, when he dies.

Many other symptoms sometimes appear from the commencement, and throughout this disease, but these are sufficient to detect it.

Treatment.—With regard to the best treatment of this disease, you must follow the directions given in Simple Inflammatory Fever, using your judgment about the remedies to be given, and the suitable time, &c. But, if a physician can be obtained, you had better lose no time, but send for one as soon as the first symptoms show themselves, and you are satisfied what disease it is.

QUINSY.

Symptoms.—This disease may be known by the patient's feeling at its commencement slight chills, which are followed by a high fever, an uneasy feeling in the throat, and pain on swallowing. In a few hours, the pain fixes itself about the tonsils (in the throat), and becomes so severe, that he swallows with great difficulty, or is entirely unable to swallow. If you look into his throat, you will see one or both of the tonsils very much swollen, and the whole surface of the throat very red and somewhat swelled. The tongue is swollen, white, and covered with a thick mucus. The face is swollen and red; the arteries of the neck beat strongly; the patient breathes with difficulty, and hears indistinctly; his voice is also indistinct, and his pulse frequent, hard, and full; his throat externally is always more or less swollen and tender.

Treatment.—Bleed immediately, and give an active purge. For this purpose, use the following :—

>   8 grains of calomel,
>   20 grains of jalap (powdered),

in one dose, mixed with syrup or honey.

You must keep the bowels well open from day to day after this, until the patient recovers. You may use for this purpose a dose or two of glauber or epsom salts every day.— (See page 32, *Cathartics*, for dose, &c.) At the same time, give the following :—

>   1 grain of tartar emetic,

dissolved in two wineglasses of water. Give a teaspoonful of this mixture every half-hour or so, until the patient becomes sick at his stomach, and keep on for some hours.

If the attack is not very severe, as soon as you have bled, rub the throat and neck with hartshorn and sweet-oil, and then apply warm poultices, and put the feet in warm water. If, however, it is severe, lose no time, but apply a fly-blister to the throat or back of the neck. After the patient has been relieved, you may let him gargle his throat with honey and warm water. Look also into the throat frequently, to see if an abscess has formed in either or both of the tonsils. If it has, pierce the tonsil with a lancet, and let out the matter.

MUMPS.

KEEP the bowels open; give gentle sweats, as flaxseed, or life-everlasting, or balm, or sage tea, and avoid taking cold. Tie a piece of flannel around the jaws. If the swelling should leave the jaws, and fall on the breasts in a woman, or the testicles in a man, but blisters under the ears, and give the patient strong sweats, and if a swelling or hardness remains after the symptoms have disappeared, rub the part with mercurial ointment or spirits of camphor.

CROUP.

Symptoms.—A dry, hoarse, and rough cough, with a change of voice, and some difficulty of breathing. This may continue for some days before the disease becomes violent. The patient generally has more or less fever from the commencement. After a while—sometimes long, sometimes short—the breathing becomes more difficult and distressing, the voice more indistinct, and sometimes destroyed; there is pain and uneasiness in the throat, and the cough is louder. The face becomes flushed, the eyes red, heavy, and protruding, the skin dry and hot, the pulse frequent, hard, and quick; the patient breathes with great difficulty. If he is not now relieved, great suffering comes on; the face becomes pale, and covered with large drops of sweat, the hands and feet cold, and many other alarming symptoms appear.

This is the usual course of the disease; sometimes, however, it comes on suddenly and with great violence, particularly in the night, and, if not immediately relieved, the patient is apt to die.

Treatment.—Bleed, without losing time, until the patient becomes sick; and if the distressing symptoms (difficulty of breathing) come on again, bleed a second and a third time if necessary. Put the patient in a warm bath, rub the throat with sweet-oil and hartshorn, or apply a strong mustard-plaster (see page 68 for directions), or wet a flannel with spirits of turpentine, and put it around his neck. Give an emetic of hippo (see page 46). If this does not puke, give another dose immediately; and if this does not act in ten or fifteen minutes, give tartar emetic, as directed, page 93. After the emetic has acted, give the following:—

  6 grains of calomel,
  3 grains of hippo or James' powder,

made into six powders. Give one of these powders every hour or two, for a child: a larger dose for a grown person. This treatment is applicable to the severe cases; but when the case is a mild one, it may not be necessary to bleed, but only to rub the throat with hartshorn and sweet-oil, give an emetic of hippo, and open the bowels with castor-oil.

After the dangerous symptoms have disappeared, use the following: A wineglassful of the seneka or large snake-root to a pint of boiling water; let it simmer on the fire fifteen or twenty minutes, and then sweeten with honey. Give a wine glass of this every hour or two.

MEASLES.

Symptoms.—A tenderness, and redness, and watery appearance, of the eyes; a watery discharge from the nose, cough and sneezing, slight chills, with flushes of heat every now and then. These are the usual symptoms, though they are not invariable. About the third or fifth day, or between them, an eruption, in the form of flea-bites, makes its appearance. This eruption soon enlarges, the number of red spots increases, they run into each other, and at last form patches of irregular shapes and sizes. Sometimes, in severe cases, the whole face swells, so as to close the eyelids. Again, on the appearance of the eruption, the fever and all of the symptoms increase, until the rash begins to fade, when they subside.

This is the *simple* form of measles, and, in general, it is only necessary to attend to these directions : Keep the bowels open with castor-oil, or some mild purge, and let the patient drink flaxseed-tea, warm, or use some diluent drinks. (See page 39.) If the fever is high, give the following :—

    1 teaspoonful of antimonial wine,
    1 tablespoonful sweet spirits of nitre.
to a wineglass of water. Give a teaspoonful every hour, and if the fever does not subside in a few hours, take a little blood.

INFLAMMATORY VARIETY OF MEASLES.

This may be known by a high fever, strong, hard, and frequent pulse, dry and very hot skin; violent, painful, harsh, and dry cough. The patient is frequently, too, out of his head during the night; his eyes are very red, and he breathes with difficulty; the rash generally very red.

Treatment.—The treatment must be according to the symptoms which appear. As a general rule, follow the directions given for the simple form, and if any particular organ or organs are the seat of the inflammation, the treatment must be the same as in other diseases attended with similar affections. Should the disease not yield to this treatment, you must send for a physician.

CONGESTIVE FORM OF MEASLES.

Symptoms.—Face pale, pulse weak and laboring, bowels confined, the patient breathes slowly and with difficulty, and the powers of life seem much depressed. There is no eruption, or it is very imperfect, and appears only in parts of the body; the feet and hands are cold, the face is shrunk, and has an uneasy expression.

Another form, or rather two forms of this disease, are noticed—the typhous and the gastric form, or where the inflammation is chiefly confined to the stomach and bowels. The typhous form so seldom occurs, that it is unnecessary to describe the treatment. In the gastric form there is not much fever; the pulse is small, weak, and very quick; the cough is distressing and almost constant. Before, and sometimes immediately after the appearance of the eruption, the patient throws up and purges violently. The tongue is brown; a severe pain in the forehead, the rash on the skin pale and indistinct, and he has short, cutting pains in his bowels, or feels a tightness and fullness in his stomach. Some other distressing symptoms also sometimes appear.

General Rule with regard to the treatment in all the forms of this disease, except the Simple.—You had better not trust your own management; but if you are compelled, adopt this plan as a general rule. For the congestive form, see directions of typhus fever, pages 86 and 87, and follow them. Where there are symptoms of inflammation and high fever, bleed moderately at first, and give warm mucilaginous drinks, as flaxseed-tea, &c., and keep the bowels gently open with castor-oil or mild purges. Use this mixture to keep the fever down: a small piece of liquorice, dissolved in a half pint of boiling water; put in one grain of tartar emetic. Give a large spoonful every two hours for a moderate-sized child.

SMALL-POX.

Symptoms.—A feeling of languor and weariness over the body, pains in the back and legs, pain in the forehead, flushes of heat, and creeping chills every now and then. After these symptoms, sickness of the stomach, vomiting, great thirst, pain in the pit of the stomach, and some soreness of the throat, are felt. As soon as the fever has risen to its height, the face and skin become dry, the tongue white, and red at the tip ; the bowels are costive, and the urine is of a deep red color, and small in quantity. Some other symptoms, more or less aggravated, show themselves, until between the third and fourth day from the commencement of the disease, when the eruption begins to make its appearance. The pimples, or pustules are first seen on the forehead, and about the mouth and nose, next on the arms, the breast, and belly, and at last, on the legs and feet. The eruption comes out entirely in about twenty-four hours. It is not necessary to describe the eruption, or the pustules, as most persons have seen them. The pustules arrive at maturity about the twelfth day, and soon after that they become drier, brown, form a crust or scab, and fall off. The scabbing always begins on the face. This is the simple or distinct variety of small-pox.

Treatment.—As soon as you are satisfied by the symptoms, that your patient has the disease, give an emetic of Hippo. (See *Emetics*, page 46.) This is not always necessary, but it is a good plan, as a general rule. If the symptoms are violent, and there is much excitement, take a little blood. In about an hour after this, open the bowels with this ;

    12 grains of calomel,
    6 grains of hippo,

made into three powders. Give one powder every three hours, until the bowels are well opened—for a grown person, less for a child. Use this also, as a drink to keep down the fever ;

    A half tablespoonful of saltpetre (powdered),
    1 grain tartar emetic,

put into a half pint of water. Give a tablespoonful of this every two hours, for a grown person. Or this ;

    2 tablespoonfuls spirits of nitre,
    1 teaspoonful of antimonial wine,

to a half pint of water : give as the other.

9

Through the whole course of the disease, keep the bowels gently open, with mild purges, and keep the skin cool with cooling drinks, such as I have recommended. Let the patient have fresh air in the room, but keep the room comfortable. Calomel is the best medicine to keep the bowels open, in doses of five grains each, and followed by a dose of castor-oil, or cream of tartar. Be careful not to purge the bowels too much.

THE CONFLUENT VARIETY OF SMALL-POX.

In this form of the disease, the patient feels very severe pains in the back and legs, during the eruption; the fever and other symptoms are generally more severe than in the simple. The tongue is sometimes covered with a dark brown, or blackish fur, and the patient is often very nervous. Although the fever is generally higher in this than in the other variety, it is sometimes of a low or typhoid character, and instead of the profuse perspiration which often occurs in the simple form, a great looseness of the bowels, just before the eruption, or when the pustules are filling, takes place in the confluent form of the disease. Again; in the confluent variety, the eruption generally appears at an earlier period of the disease, than in the simple; the pustules sometimes coming out on the second day, though sometimes not until the fifth.

In confluent small-pox, the pustules are generally of an irregular shape, and not so elevated as in the other. The face and hands are much more swelled, the throat more sore, and the spittle flows from the mouth more freely. This is not *always* the case, however. When the pustules fill, the fever increases.

About the eighth or ninth day, from the commencement of the eruption, the matter comes out of the pustules, and becomes hard on the skin, and then falls off in flakes, or crusts, leaving sometimes, deep pits or furrows on the face. Sometimes this form makes its attacks very violently, and is highly inflammatory and dangerous, the eyes become very red, and various alarming symptoms appear.

Again, in the simple variety, we sometimes see the disease of a low or typhoid character. The patient is very weak and much prostrated, and various bad symptoms, showing nervous derangement, appear. Sometimes the eruption comes out slowly and imperfectly, and disappears quickly. This is always dangerous. Sometimes the disease is of a malignant or putrid character. particularly the confluent variety; the heat of the skin is burning, the perspiration offensive; frequently the bowels are very loose, and the passages watery; the pustules look dark, and are filled with a bloody humor, and many other disgusting symptoms appear.

These are the usual symptoms of this disease, and such the usual course; but sometimes we see other symptoms, and the disease is irregular in its course, and different in its general character.

With regard to the treatment, as a rule, follow the directions on page 97, and when you see other symptoms, treat them according to your judgment.

In order to prevent the disease from spreading on plantations and in other places, attend to these directions. Keep the patients to themselves, and do not allow others to go and see them, or their nurses to attend on any who have not the disease. When they have recovered, burn all the bedding and clothing which they have been using; remove them to another house (by themselves), and smoke out the house in which they have been, well, with tar or pine-wood; then give it a thick coat of whitewash, inside and outside. Be careful when you come from visiting a patient, to smoke yourself (that is, your clothes), so as not to carry the disease into another house. By attention to these directions, the disease can be prevented from spreading on the largest plantations. I have, myself, in this way, prevented it from spreading on several plantations, where the houses were close together.

VARIOLOID, OR MODIFIED SMALL-POX.

Symptoms.—In this disease, the fever is generally so mild as to be scarcely perceptible, though it is sometimes very violent, but it always ceases when the eruption comes out. The eruption generally appears, at first, in the form of small pimples, many of which dry off without becoming larger. Frequently, however, they grow into pustules, which contain a watery humor, and about the third or fourth day, burst, or dry up. Frequently, also, these pustules are surrounded by a red or reddish mark. Again; these pustules are frequently filled with a thick humor, have a depression or pit in their centre, and on the third or fourth day, change into thin, dark scabs, and about the sixth or seventh day after the appearance of the eruption, fall off. They sometimes, however, remain until the tenth or twelfth day. These pustules sometimes also assume other appearances, and often look so much like those of the genuine or simple small-pox, that it is difficult to distinguish them ; and sometimes the eruption is so thick as to resemble confluent small-pox.

The pustules in varioloid seldom or never leave a pit, unless the scabs remain a long time before they fall off, though sometimes they leave excrescences like warts. This disease is very irregular in its course and symptoms, according to the age and condition of the patient.

Treatment.—If the eruption is slow in coming out, give an emetic of hippo (see *Emetics,* page 46), and treat the disease in the same manner as measles, page 95.

INFLAMMATION OF THE BRAIN, OR PHRENSY.

Symptoms.—Pain and fulness in the head, and, generally, sick stomach and puking. The eyes become red and sparkling, the face flushed, and the patient complains of an uneasy feeling along his back. The patient also soon gets out of his head, and in a short time becomes furious. At first, the pulse is strong and full, but soon becomes small, and feels tight, like a cord, and sometimes stops every now and then. Frequently the patient has symptoms of jaundice, and derangement of the liver.

Treatment.—Bleed immediately, and let the blood flow until the patient is sick at his stomach. If he is not relieved by one bleeding, bleed again and again, from time to time. Cut the hair short, or shave the head, and apply a bladder half full of cold water, with a piece of ice in it, if it can be had. Keep a bladder constantly to the top of the head. If he is a grown person, give him ten grains of calomel and four hours afterward, a dose of Epsom or glauber salts (see *Cathartics*, pages 32 and 34); less for a child, &c. Cup the temples, or put leeches to them. Remember the bowels must be kept open during the whole course of the disease; the patient ought to have a passage about every six hours, until he is better, and then they must be kept gently open. Be careful not to salivate the patient. (For medicines to act on the bowels, see *Cathartics*, from page 31.) Put a blister on the back of the neck, and keep putting them on as soon as the place heals, throughout the course of the disease. Use this, also, from the commencement, until the patient is decidedly better;

    1 teaspoonful of saltpetre (powdered),
    1 grain of tartar emetic, or a papspoonful of antimonial wine,

in a half pint of water. Give a tablespoonful of this every two hours. Remember, also, to keep the patient's head raised. When the patient is recovering, give this;

    10 grains of saltpetre,
    ½ grain of digitalis (powder),

every two or three hours. You may continue or stop this, from time to time, at discretion. If you use the tincture of digitalis, take a teaspoonful and put it and the saltpetre into a half pint of water, and give a tablespoonful. Be careful to keep the room dark and quiet; and, as long as the patient has fever or pain in the head, he must have nothing for nourishment but toast-water. Steep the toasted bread in hot water, and give the water.

ACUTE DROPSY IN THE BRAIN.

Symptoms.—The patient is wakeful at night, peevish, and can not bear a strong light. Small children cry frequently without any cause, start often in their sleep, and frequently scream violently. Those at the breast when awake, often start suddenly, or at the slightest noise, and scream as if they felt a sudden pain. These symptoms may show themselves for some time, and the child (for this disease occurs much more frequently in children), gradually got better; more frequently, however, they continue until the disease runs into the *second,*

or inflammatory stage, which may be known by the following
symptoms; shooting pains in the head, and pains in the bowels; increased restlessness and irritability of temper; irritated,
quick, tight, and active pulse; the face expressive of uneasiness
and suffering; a flush in one or both cheeks, the eyelids half
closed, and the eyebrows frowning. The discharges from the
bowels, which are sometimes costive and sometimes loose, are
of an unnatural color. These symptoms increase as the disease advances. Children affected with this disease, frequently put their hands to their foreheads. At this time, also,
puking is apt to come on, especially when the child sits up.
You will generally notice, that in an advanced stage of this
disease, the patient sighs often, and children are constantly
stretching out their arms, which tremble very much, as they
lay on the bed, and putting them to their heads. The skin
is generally dry, and warmer than natural, the tongue clean,
with pale edges, or covered with a thin white fur. There is,
generally, too, delirium, but not violent, and not continued.

These are the usual symptoms which characterize this
disease, and the most important which it is requisite to notice; several others appear, and there are frequently devia-
tions from peculiar circumstances, but my limits will not per-
mit me to become particular.

The Third Stage.—After these symptoms just described
have lasted some time, water on the brain is formed, which
you may know by the following symptoms. The delirium is
more constant, the countenance exhibits the aspect of stupor
and surprise, the eyes are watery and reddish, and turned up
under the upper eyelids during sleep. The patient is constantly sleepy, inattentive to what is passing around him, and
when aroused quickly, relapses into stupor. These symptoms continue or increase, until the patient becomes para-
lyzed in one side, and unable to raise the eyelids without
moving the muscles of the forehead. Sometimes the patient
appears suddenly better, but he soon relapses.

This disease does not come on always in the manner I have
described; but after some appearances of ill health, such as
fretfulness, bad breath, swelled upper lip, puffed belly, grinding
the teeth during sleep, &c., the water suddenly forms on the
brain. Sometimes, even these symptoms do not precede it.
You will generally observe that in the latter stages of this
disease, the passages are dark green, like chopped spinage.

Treatment.—In the commencement of the disease, give one or two grains of calomel or blue pill every evening, followed next morning with a small dose of Epsom salts, powdered rhubarb, or castor-oil (see *Cathartics*, pages 32 and 33), for a child of five years old or younger. Continue this treatment from day to day, until the passages look natural. Give the patient, as nourishment, rice or corn gruel, arrow-root, boiled milk, thin beef or chicken water, and be careful to give them a little at a time. As soon as the *inflammatory* stage comes on, take blood carefully, according to the pulse. If it is a child, put leeches to the temples and behind the ears; if a grown person, cup the temples. The bowels must be kept open, and the best medicines are calomel, followed by castor-oil, senna, or Epsom salts. After the bowels have been well opened, at first keep them open by giving two grains of calomel every three hours, during the day, until the patient takes ten grains, if a grown person; half for a child five or six years old. You must regulate your purges by the bowels. When the passages are large and offensive, give full doses until they are natural; but generally give moderate doses, so as not to purge too much. If the child has worms, you must give (cautiously) worm medicines at the same time. (See *Anthelmintics*, pages 25 and 26: read the table and see directions.) If the stomach is very irritable, give this:—

    1 grain of calomel,
    3 grains of hippo,

made into six powders. Give one powder every half-hour, until the puking is checked. If the inflammation remains high and obstinate, give this:-

    6 grains of calomel,
    6 grains of James' powder,

made into six powders; give one powder every hour, for a grown person. After the inflammation and determination to the head have been subdued, if the patient is not better, put a blister to the back of the neck, bladders of cold water to the head, and salivate by rubbing mercurial ointment in the groin and arm-pits, and even over the whole body, if necessary.

    With regard to the other disease of ths brain, viz., *softening of the brain*, I will only remark that, as it is not of every-day occurrence, it is not necessary to describe it; but the treatment is very similar to that for inflammation of the brain, or phrensy.

ACUTE INFLAMMATION OF THE STOMACH.

Symptoms.—Frequent and painful puking after drinking warm fluids; a great thirst for cool drinks, and great aversion to warm; sometimes a burning and shooting pain in the stomach, or tenderness of the stomach, sickness, and puking. Sometimes delirium, low spirits, weakness; pulse at first somewhat full, but soon becomes quick, small, tight—sometimes so as to be scarcely felt. The face has a look of great suffering and despair. When the stomach is alone inflamed, the bowels are costive; but when one of the large bowels are so also, diarrhœa, straining, and dysentery, come on; dry and generally hot skin; tongue commonly clean and red, or with a thick white fur along the middle, with red and rough edges.

These are the usual and most important symptoms, but they do not always occur, and the disease may progress and become fatal without exhibiting them.

Be careful not to confound this disease with the cramp, or wind in the bowels. For in the one, the pulse is small and quick, the pain is steady, the patient lies constantly on his back, which is not the case in cramp.

Treatment.—Bleed immediately, until the patient feels it. Next put leeches over the stomach, or cup it; after these are removed, put on a large blister.—(See page 69, *Fly-Blister*.) Dress the blister with mercurial ointment, spread on a rag. Let the patient drink freely of flaxseed-tea (cool), or gum-Arabic in water, or orange-juice in water. Keep the bowels open with clysters in this way:—

    2 wineglasses of castor-oil,
    1 tablespoonful of Castile soap (scraped),
    ½ pint of flaxseed-tea,

mixed together. After the patient has been well bled, and his bowels well opened, give this:—

    4 grains of calomel,
    4 grains of powdered opium,

made into four pills. Give one every three hours during the day. When the patient is getting better, be careful to give him no solid food.

CHRONIC INFLAMMATION OF THE STOMACH.

Symptoms.—Acid stomach, and eructation, slight pains about the stomach occasionally, wind in the bowels, and a sense of weight or oppression about the stomach after eating. The patient's appetite is often irregular, sometimes craving and sometimes abhorring food ; he feels easier when the stomach is empty, but relaxed and discontented. The symptoms generally mark the early stages of the disease, but as it advances, the part above the stomach becomes puffed and somewhat tender to the touch, and the patient is apt to become sick, or to throw up an hour or so after eating. The pain in the stomach is generally in one spot, and shooting or stinging. Some patients complain of a ball, and others of a feeling as if a bar was across their stomach, preventing the food from passing. Sometimes they throw up a quantity of white glairy fluid. There is generally a disgust for food ; and generally the patient is costive from the commencement of the disease ; but when the disease is advanced, looseness of the bowels, straining, and griping, come on, and the passages are slimy and bloody. The tongue is generally clean, smooth, and of a bright-red color, or with raised spots, like a strawberry, having deep seams or fissures ; or, again, with a streak of brown fur along the middle, and its edges clean and red ; the pulse generally quick and somewhat corded, though not always, at the commencement of the disease ; and when the disease is far advanced, it is hard, small, and quick.

These are the usual symptoms of this disease. It may, however, progress to a dangerous stage without showing any serious symptoms. And it is sometimes very irregular in its course, and exhibits symptoms different from these, or some others besides.

Treatment.—Pay great attention to the patient's food : nothing irritating must be eaten or drank. Give him boiled barley, rice or corn gruel, arrow-root, sago, boiled milk, jellies, &c., but no solid food. Let him drink flaxseed-tea and such drinks as are under the head of diluents.—(See p. 39.) If the case is obstinate, put leeches or cups to the stomach, and when these are removed, apply a blister.—(See *Fly-Blisters*, page 69.) Or you may rub the part over the stomach with tartar-emetic ointment, until pimples are brought out. Continue this treatment from time to time.

Give this also:—

4 grains of the extract of hyosciamus (henbane),
½ grain of sulphate of morphine,
2 grains of sulphate of iron,

rubbed together and divided into four parts. Give one part every six hours during the day and night. This is also good:

1 teaspoonful balsam Copaiva,
30 drops of the acet. tincture of opium,
½ wineglass of lemon-syrup,
1 teaspoonful of gum-Arabic (powdered),

to one half pint of water. Give a tablespoonful of this mixture in the morning, and one in the evening. You may give two or three grains also of Dover's powder every night, when the patient is in bed. Lastly, keep the bowels open well by giving a clyster once or twice a day.—(See page 70.) But it is dangerous to give medicine by the mouth.

ACUTE INFLAMMATION OF THE BOWELS.

Symptoms.—An uneasy feeling in some part of the belly, and, after some time, a burning pain, generally about the navel; bowels almost always obstinately costive—sometimes, but very seldom, dysentery and straining; generally sickness at the stomach, and violent puking, and the patient sometimes throws up dung; tongue dry, and generally with a white fur, or with a streak of brown fur along the middle, and pale-red edges; great thirst, urine highly colored and small quantity, and pain and difficulty in making water; forehead and palms of the hands generally moist, the rest of the body hot and dry. He breathes short, and raises his chest up and down; pulse small, feels tight and quick. The patient lies on his back, with his knees drawn up and his shoulders raised, so as not to stretch the muscles of his belly. Sometimes the disease begins with these symptoms: a slight chill, followed by a fever or excitement, then a sinking of the whole body; the feet and hands cold, and lastly damp; great weakness, face as pale as death, hands and fingers mottled, belly tight and swelled, and the pulse weak, soft, and undulating; lastly, the bowels puffed with a great quantity of wind. Be careful not to confound this disease with colic, as the patient lies quiet, instead of rolling and tossing about as in colic.

Treatment.—Bleed immediately, until the patient feels sick, and take a little blood every now and then, when the pulse indicates it, until the violence of the inflammation is subdued. Then apply leeches or cups over the stomach. Keep the bowels open with mild cathartics or laxatives. At the commencement of the disease, use injections of this kind, to open the bowels, before you give the purgative medicines :—

One pint of boiling water poured on a wineglassful of flaxseed ; pour off the water, and give injections with it.

When you have reduced the inflammation by bleeding, leeching, and injections, as directed, give this :—

    5 or 8 grains of calomel,
    2 grains of opium (powdered),

made into one powder, and given every two hours, until the pain in the belly is relieved, and the skin becomes soft ; then give a wineglassful of castor-oil, and if this does not purge out the bowels well, give a half-wineglassful of the same every two hours, until it does. If, again, you can not produce purging in this way, give this injection :—

    1 pint of flaxseed-tea (warm),
    A wineglassful of the oil of turpentine,
    With the whites of two eggs.

Throw this injection up the bowels, and then give two grains of powdered opium, in one dose, and let the patient go to sleep. If the patient is not decidedly better now, put a blister over the belly, or warm poultices of cornmeal, boiled, with a teaspoonful of powdered opium in each poultice. When all these have been resorted to without effect, try this :

    A teaspoonful of snuff,
    To 1 pint of water.

Give this in two injections. This disease sometimes terminates in mortification of the bowels. When this is about to take place, you will notice these symptoms : the pain generally ceases, the pulse becomes very small and weak, the hands and feet are very cold, and great weakness of the whole body. You must not, however, give up when you observe these symptoms, but stimulate with good wine, and give freely

of the mucilaginous drinks, if the stomach can bear them.—
(See *Demulcents*, page 40.)

When the patient is recovering, give nothing but the mildest food, so as not to irritate the bowels; and when the bowels (as they are apt to be) are filled with wind, rub the belly with a flesh-brush, or use injections, with a little mint-water or asafœtida in them.

ACUTE INFLAMMATION OF THE LINING MEMBRANE OF THE BOWELS.

This disease is of two forms. First, where the inflammation is seated in the large bowels, or rather in what is called the duodenum. When this is the case, you will observe the following—

Symptoms.—The whole surface of the body frequently jaundiced, appetite bad, bitter taste in the mouth, tongue covered generally with a whitish fur; water of a high color, and small in quantity; not much pain in the bowels; headache, bowels sluggish, but may be moved by gentle purges and clysters. The pulse feels like a cord, and generally fuller than in inflammation of the stomach.

The second form is where the disease is confined to the small intestines, and may be known by the following—

Symptoms.—The bowels sometimes loose, or easily moved, and the passages slimy; the belly hard and tender; the tongue has a white or light-brown fur along the middle, and its edges and tip are of a bright color; irritable stomach generally, and a slight burning pain, and a feeling of weight about the navel.

The treatment of these two forms of disease which I have just described does not differ materially from that of acute inflammation of the bowels (page 107).

DYSENTERY.

THIS disease is the same as that just described, only located in two of the lower large bowels, namely, the colon and the rectum.

Symptoms.—Wandering pains in the bowels and occasionally looseness, but usually costiveness, loss of appetite, bad taste in the mouth, sick stomach, chills, with flushes of heat every now and then, thirst and dry skin, low pulse. Sometimes sudden griping comes on, with slimy and bloody passages, attended with great straining. Frequently, also, there is pain and difficulty in passing water. In advanced stages of the disease, the passages often have a very disagreeable smell. The tongue is at first generally covered with a white fur, which, as the diseases advances, becomes brown, rough, and dry, with the edges red and moist. When the disease lasts a long time, or the inflammation is not of an acute character, the edges and tip of the tongue are usually clean, smooth, and red, and sometimes the whole tongue is smooth, clean, and red, like raw flesh. The passages, generally, contain no bile. In aggravated forms of this disease, many other symptoms may appear, and the disease may deviate from the course which I have described; but you will find no difficulty in detecting it, if you pay attention to them.

Treatment.—Attention to the disease at its commencement, is of the utmost importance. As a general rule, whenever the pulse is firm and quick, or hard and frequent, bleed. If, however, the fever is not high, but of a low, or typhoid character, do not bleed. Give an emetic of hippo at the commencement of the disease.—(See page 46.) This is not always necessary ; but if the tongue has a brown fur along the middle, or there is sick stomach and puking of bile, give it. Next, about two hours after the emetic, give this:—10 or 12 grains of calomel, made into two powders. Give one powder two hours after the other (for a grown person), and three or four hours after the last powder, give a dose of castor oil and laudanum.—(See page 71.) If the medicine does not produce good passages, but griping and straining, give a dose of opium (gum).—(See page 29.) When the disease is, in a measure subdued, give this:—

      6 grains of calomel,

      24 grains of Dover's powder,

10

made into six or eight powders, Give one powder every three hours, until the griping is checked. Or this:—

 2 grains of calomel,

 2 grains James' powder (best),

 1 grain powdered opium,

made into eight powders; give one every two or three hours.

————

CHRONIC DYSENTERY.

When the symptoms of inflammation have disappeared, and the discharge from the bowels is still obstinate, showing that the discharge has become *chronic dysentery*, you must give calomel until you see a slime on the tongue, and the passages look good. Use this:—

 12 grains calomel,

 2 grains of powdered opium,

made into six pills; give one pill every three hours. Give also this:—

 1 pint of flaxseed tea (warm),

 ½ grain of sulphate of morphine.

Give a wineglassful of this every hour. Let the patient take free also, for nourishment, chicken water, and such medicines as are mentioned in page 39 (*Diluents*). You must also use anodyne clysters (see page 70), and emollient clysters, such as flaxseed and starch (see page 70). If, after all these, the disease is still obstinately continued, give this:—

 1 teaspoonful of powdered gum arabic,

 ½ wineglassful balsam copaiva,

 2 teaspoonfuls of white sugar,

 1 teaspoonful of laudanum,

 In a half-pint of water.

Give a tablespoonful of this mixture every two or three hours. Or, you may try this:—

 3 grains of Dover's powders,

 10 grains crab's-eyes,

made into one powder. Give a powder every three or four hours.

As a last resort, when all these have failed, salivate the patient with this :—

    6 grains of calomel,
    1 grain of sulph. morphine,

made into three pills or powders ; give one every three hours. Or this :—

    12 grains blue pill,
    2 grains morphine,
    5 grains compound extract of colocynth,

made into four pills ; give one pill every three hours. When the patient is getting better, he must take no solid food, but such things as are mentioned, page 39 (*Diluents*). As a drink, give this—a wineglassful of the bark of slippery-elm (powder) pour on it a pint of boiling water, and give a wineglassful every hour, when cool.

CHRONIC INFLAMMATION OF THE MUCOUS MEMBRANE OF THE BOWELS.

WHENEVER you hear people talking of marasmus, liver complaint, dyspepsia, &c., you may conclude that they mean this disease; as its symptoms are rather obscure, and it is apt to be mistaken for other complaints. You may know it, however, by the following

Symptoms.—Pain and a soreness about the bowels whenever the patient coughs and sneezes ; or pressure is made on his bowels : languor and weakness of the body ; generally cold hands and feet, flushed cheeks, slight fever in the evening, a burning in the palms of the hands and soles of the feet ; a small, weak, sharp or corded pulse : usually a pain, like colic, in the bowels after eating ; sometimes diarrhœa, and sometimes costiveness ; appetite very variable. When the disease has lasted a long time, the patient feels uneasy, after eating, until he obtains a passage, and the food which comes away, looks half digested. The patient wastes away rapidly now. In children, as the limbs shrivel, the belly becomes large. Considerable straining, and the discharges from the bowels are sometimes slimy and small in quantity, mixed with the natural passes, sometimes like bloody matter; sometimes watery and in quantity, and sometimes dark, or whitish, having pieces of food undigested in them. Skin dry, sallow or dingy, tongue generally smooth and red at the edges, with a brown streak along the middle.

Treatment.—You must pay great attention to the patient's food; he must not eat any solid food, but such as these; arrow-root, prepared barley, rice boiled soft with boiled milk; he may occasionally take a soft boiled egg. Keep the bowels gently open with a dose of castor oil and ten drops of laudanum, but do not give active purges. If the disease remains obstinate, leech and cup, and even blister the belly, and when the place has healed, put on a tight flannel bandage around the belly. You may give these powders, also, occasionally

> 25 grains of Dover's powder,
> 1 grain of calomel,

made into 8 powders; give one powder every five or six hours, during the day. Or this:—

> $\frac{1}{2}$ wineglassful of the spirits of turpentine,
> 1 teaspoonful of laudanum,
> 1 tablespoonful of white sugar,

rubbed up with the white of an egg, to 3 wineglasses of water; mix them together and give a teaspoonful three or four times during the day. You may try five or six drops of balsam copaiva every day, if these fail.

ACUTE INFLAMMATION OF THE LIVER.

Symptoms.—Slight febrile symptoms, a feeling of tightness in the right side and the pit of the stomach. There is very often, too, pain in the chest, shoulder, or collar-bone. Pain in the right side, on pressure. Generally a dry cough, and difficulty of breathing, sometimes sick stomach and puking of bile. The whites of the eyes, and skin about the breast, face and neck, somewhat yellow. Urine deep yellowish brown, with bile in it; great thirst, hot and dry skin; full, active and firm pulse; bowels generally costive. These are the usual symptoms, when the inflammation is seated in the substance of the liver, but when it is merely on the surface, the pulse is small, tight, and quick; tongue covered with a white or thick yellowish fur, or smooth and glossy, having fissures or furrows, and appears raised in some places. The bowels are sometimes, but not often, loose, and much griping, as in dysentery.

This disease, when it continues beyond the sixth or seventh day, is apt to produce abscess of the liver. When this has occurred, the pain in the side is lessened, and instead, there is a sensation of weight and throbbing, with chills at times, sweats at night, a feeling or sinking or oppression in the chest, and a crawling of the skin, skin clammy. Sometimes the abscess opens outward, and you may let out the matter with a lancet or knife. Sometimes it points internally, and the matter is discharged through the bowels or lungs. Be careful not to confound this disease with inflammation of the stomach.

Treatment.—Bleed until the pulse is evidently affected, then give 15 or 20 grains of calomel, in one dose, and about two hours afterward, a wineglass of castor oil. If one bleeding does not succeed, repeat it several times in the course of the first few days, then apply leeches over the stomach and liver. Keep the bowels well open, by giving 8 or 10 grains of calomel, twice or three times a day, and if the bowels are not opened by this, give a small dose of Epsom or glauber salts, two hours after each dose, until they are (see pages 32 and 34, for *doses*, &c), or castor oil. After you have, in a measure, reduced the inflammation by bleeding, and opened the bowels well, as directed, put blisters over the liver (that is, over the short ribs on the right side), and keep the bowels open by giving these powders:—

    3 grains of calomel,
    3 grains of antimonial powder,
    1 grain of powdered opium,

made into one powder, and given every five hours, until the gums are a little sore. If these powders do not keep the bowels well open, you must give a dose of castor oil or Epsom salts between them every now and then. Remember that blisters must be kept constantly over the liver—as fast as one heals sufficiently, put on another. Give this, also:—

    2 grains of antimonial powder,
    2 grains of saltpetre (powdered),
10*

every four hours, and let the patient drink warm flaxseed tea, or gum water; if these powders irritate the stomach, stop them. When an abscess has formed in the liver, keep the bowels well open by 5 or 6 grains of calomel every now and then, followed in four hours by a dose of castor-oil or Epsom salts, and bathe the patient's feet and hands in this mixture: one half a wineglass of nitric and muriatic acid, mixed in one gallon of warm water.

And let the patient take this: a teaspoonful of these acids to a tumbler of water. Give a wineglassful (sucked through a quill), every three hours during the day.

CHRONIC INFLAMMATION OF THE LIVER.

Symptoms.—This disease frequently remains as a consequence of the acute form, but sometimes it comes like any other disease. When it comes on, from whatever cause, you will observe these

Symptoms.—Acid, and sometimes sick stomach and puking; bad appetite, indigestion, wind, and sometimes slight pains in the bowels, and a feeling of fullness about the stomach.— Sometimes the patient feels a slight dull pain and weight in the right side, about the short ribs; and frequently a pain in the right shoulder. The pain in the right side, however, is frequently not felt, unless the part is pressed upon, when the patient feels an uneasiness and tightness there. The face looks thin and sickly. The whites of the eyes, skin of the face, neck and heart yellowish. Bowels generally costive, but sometimes loose, and the passages are disagreeable, small, dark, slimy, and greenish, or muddy and watery. Water colored with bile, and burns high up the bladder when it is passed. Tongue generally dry and white, a bitter and disagreeable taste in the mouth; dry, harsh skin. Sometimes a dry cough and difficulty of breathing. This disease is very common among those who live in swamps and unhealthy parts.

Treatment.—Put leeches or cups over the liver, and when

these are removed, put on, from time to time, warm, soft poul-tices.—(See pages 68 and 69.) Open the bowels gently with castor oil, or with this :—

      6 grains of calomel,
      10 grains of rhubarb,
      2 grains of James' powders,

given at one dose, in syrup or honey. Then use this :—

      4 grains of blue pill,
      1 grain of the comp. extract of colocynth, or of the
          extract of conium, or hyosciamus,

if you can get them, made into one pill. Give a pill three times a day, from day to day, until you find the gums a little sore, then stop until the gums are well, and go on again as before, until the disease is cured, but be careful not to salivate. While you are giving these pills, you must keep the bowels gently open, by giving, every now and then, a small·dose of Epsom or glauber salts, or rhubarb (powder).—(See pages 32, 34, and 33.) In connexion with the other remedies, you may use this, to give tone to the stomach, and keep the bowels in a good state :—

      2 teaspoonfuls of the tincture gentian,
      1 teaspoonful of the carbonate of soda,
      30 drops.of nitric acid,

mixed with a half-pint of the decoction of sarsaparilla, which last is made thus. Take as much of the root of the sarsapa-rilla (broken up), as will get into a very small tumbler, put this into a pan and pour a pint of water on it; boil this down to a half-pint, and mix it. Give a tablespoonful of this mix-ture every morning, noon, and evening. Bathe the feet as directed in page 68. If the disease remains obstinate, rub the part over the liver with this :—

      1 teaspoonful of white precipitate, rubbed up with a
          tablespoonful of lard.

Rub this over the liver two or three times a day, until pustules come out.

The patient must be kept in a dry atmosphere and a comfortable room—wear warm clothing, avoid taking cold, and eat nothing but the most wholesome food.

ACUTE INFLAMMATION OF THE SPLEEN.

This disease is not very common, but the symptoms are, a heavy pain under the false ribs of the left side, which is much increased when pressed upon; sometimes a pain under the right shoulder-blade, and the place looks a little swollen. Frequently, also a burning in the stomach, sickness and giddiness, and other bad feelings, particularly when the patient sits up in bed; skin and eyes yellowish, and water colored with bile. Notice these symptoms, as you are apt to mistake this disease for inflammation of the liver.

Treatment.—Bleed until the pulse is reduced, then purge out the bowels in the same manner as in acute inflammation of the bowels (page 107). After the bowels have been well purged out, put the patient into a warm bath, and attend to the directions, generally, in pages 107 and 108.

CHRONIC INFLAMMATION OF THE SPLEEN.

Symptoms.—A sickly and gloomy countenance, fretful temper, uneasy and painful feelings at times, and the patient can not lie on the left side; sometimes the patient throws up blood.

Treatment.—Leech or cup the part over the spleen, which is on the left side, under the short ribs; and when this is done, rub the place with tartar emetic ointment, until pustules come out; and put the patient into a warm bath every now and then. Keep the bowels constantly open by giving these pills;

4 grains of blue pill,
1 grain of extract of hyosciamus,

made into one pill; give a pill every morning and evening, until the gums are sore, then stop and go on again, until the disease is cured. You may give this also;

1 grain of James' powder,
3 grains of saltpetre.

Give this every night and morning, or very small doses of tartar emetic, say one fourth of a grain, at a dose. You may use, also, every now and then, some of the medicines in pages 35 to 38 (*Diaphoretics*).

ENLARGEMENT AND INDURATION OF THE SPLEEN.

This is very apt to occur from intermitting fever, and is common among those who live on swamps, marshes, and in unhealthy parts of the country.

Symptoms.—This disease may be known by a large swelling on the left side, about the short ribs, which sometimes rises and falls. Very often, too, the skin is discolored in this place, and you will see what is well known as the *fever cake.*

Treatment.—Give this;

1 tablespoonful of Peruvian bark (powdered),
1 teaspoonful of rhubarb (powder),
1 teaspoonful of sal-ammoniac (powdered),

rubbed together, and made into four powders. Give one powder every two hours during the day. Give this, also, as a drink;

1 grain of tartar emetic,
2 quarts of warm flaxseed tea.

Give a wineglassful every two or three hours during the day, for eight days or so. Keep the bowels constantly open with this;

2 grains of blue pill,
1 grain of antimonial powder,

made into one pill. Give a pill every night and morning, and if they do not keep the bowels open sufficiently, give a dose of some mild purge, as Epsom salts, rhubarb, or castor oil, every now and then. Put the patient into a warm bath every night, and rub the spleen frequently with a brush, and put a tight flannel bandage around his belly, and let him wear it. If the disease is obstinate, you may give this; 8 or 10 drops of the tincture of iodime, three times a day, or rub the part over the spleen frequently with the iodine ointment.

———

ACUTE INFLAMMATION OF THE MEMBRANE WHICH SURROUNDS ALL THE BOWELS OF THE ABDOMEN —CALLED THE PERITONEUM.

Symptoms.—Creeping chills, with flushes of heat every now and then, weariness of the body, and pain in the limbs. Frequently sharp pain in some part of the belly, which, after remaining in one spot for a short time, spreads over the whole or most of the belly. This is not always the case, for sometimes, in the most severe cases, there is no pain, but only a little uneasiness about the bowels.; and sometimes the pain flies about from one place to another in the bowels. There is always much pain when you press on the belly ; and the patient will lie on his back, with his knees and shoulders raised to prevent the covering from pressing on his bowels. Weight and uneasiness about the stomach, and headache. Pulse frequent, and somewhat hard and small, and sometimes, but very seldom, full. Face generally pale, sharp, and anxious; bowels costive; tongue moist, and at first covered with a thin white fur, and the edges red, as the disease advances. Urine small in quantity, and sometimes none at all. Restlessness, short, quick, painful, and difficult breathing. Generally the belly swells, and becomes tight in about twenty-four hours after the disease has commenced. When this disease occurs in females, just after their confinement, it is called *puerperal* fever, and the patient sinks much sooner than when it occurs in other patients.

This disease is generally very rapid in its course, and may end in death in a few days, or even hours ; or sometimes, but not often, in mortification; or the patient may get better, or, lastly, it may end in chronic peritonitis. When it ends in mortification, the pain in the bowels suddenly ceases, the patient becomes very weak, his pulse very small and quick, and frequently stops every now and then ; the hands and feet become cold and clammy, &c. When you see these symptoms the case is hopeless.

Treatment.—Bleed immediately until the patient is sick, and if the pain and fever come on again, bleed a second, or even a third time, if necessary ; but remember, never bleed after the first twenty-four hours, as it is dangerous.

When you find that the fever and inflammation have been subdued, in a measure, by the bleeding, put leeches, if you can get them, all over the belly; if not, cup the belly in several places, and after the leeches or cups come off, keep flannels, wrung out in warm water, constantly applied all over the belly. As soon as you find the pain and tenderness in the bowels relieved in a measure, give this (if a grown person) ;

> 10 grains of calomel,
> 20 grains of jalap,

rubbed up and made into two powders. Give one powder an hour after the other, and in two hours after the last powder, if the bowels are not open, give this;

A large wineglass of castor oil,

A tablespoonful of spirits of turpentine;

mix them, and divide them into two doses. Give one dose, and if it does not purge in two hours, give the other. If, after you have bled and purged out the patient well, the belly is still tender and painful when you press it, put a blister over it, and instead of using oil and wax, use mercurial ointment to dress the blister with. When the violence of the inflammation appears to have been subdued, give this;

3 grains of calomel,

1 grain of powdered opium,

made into one powder. Give a powder every three or four hours during the day, until the patient is decidedly better, then use this;—one grain of powdered digitalis, in a little honey or syrup, every two or three hours, until the pulse becomes soft and natural. Sometimes when the patient appears to be doing well, particularly a female, just after childbirth, they will suddenly sink and become very weak, and all, or most, of the symptoms of mortification, as I have described, will suddenly appear. When you see this, give wine immediately, a glass four or five times a day, and if it does not quickly rouse the patient, give this;

3 grains of gum camphor,

1 grain of powdered opium,

rubbed together with a little white sugar, and made into one powder. Give a powder every three or four hours during the day, and night, at intervals of three hours, and continue this until the patient is restored. When the patient is getting better, take great care that he eats nothing but thin rice gruel or barley, and that he does not take cold.

CHRONIC INFLAMMATION OF THE MEMBRANE WHICH SURROUNDS ALL THE BOWELS OF THE ABDOMEN —CALLED THE PERITONEUM.

Tuis disease is very insidious in its attack, and frequently becomes dangerous before it is suspected. It generally occurs as a consequence of the acute form, and may be known by these

Symptoms.—The belly feels tight, rather than painful, particularly when the bowels are costive; and the patient sometimes complains of a feeling, as if a ball was rolling about in his bowels. There is sometimes a slight pain in the belly, which leaves and returns. But most frequently there is a soreness and uneasiness about the navel, when the belly is pressed upon, or the patient coughs and sneezes, and sometimes a pricking sensation about the lower part of the belly, after exercise or exertion. But the belly never feels tight to the hand, when pressed upon, as in the acute form; but the skin feels loose, while you can feel as if there was a tight bandage underneath. Pulse not much altered, except about evening, or when the disease is far advanced, and then it is quick and small. Face and skin generally pale and sickly. After this disease has lasted sometime, water is apt to be formed on the bowels. You must be very careful to notice the symptoms of this disease, as they are apt to escape notice, or puzzle even physicians.

Treatment.—Put leeches or cups over the whole belly, and when these are removed, dress the place with mercurial ointment. Open the bowels and keep them constantly open by castor oil, cream of tartar, or mild purges, and give one of these powders every night and morning;

      3 grains of calomel,
      2 grains of Doyer's powders.

But the food which the patient uses, is of more importance in the cure of this disease than medicine. The patient must positively take only as much nourishment as is absolutely necessary for sustenance, and that of the lightest kind, as soft boiled rice, gruel, &c.

INFLAMMATION OF THE KIDNEYS.

This disease may be produced by cold or by blows, strains, gravel, and irritating substances, rheumatism, or some disease settling on the kidneys. When it comes on in females, the symptoms are like those of other complaints caused by cold, su h as chills, with flushes of heat every now and then, and when the fever comes on, there is pain in the loins. But when it proceeds from the other causes which I have mentioned, these are the

Symptoms.—A deep-seated, severe pain in the loin, on one or both sides, which is not much increased by pressure, but is by any sudden jerk or jar of the body. Sometimes the pain darts down to one testicle, and a numbness is felt in the thigh of that side. There is very little water passed, and that high colored, and, sometimes, tinged with blood, and great desire to pass it. Bowels costive, frequently sick stomach, and puking, and severe wind pains in the bowels. Sometimes a dull pain begins low down, and moves slowly up to the back. The skin generally hot and dry, the pulse hard, full, and quick, in the beginning, afterward small and quick. This disease does not last longer than the seventh day, without an abscess in the kidney, or the inflammation subsiding. When an abscess is forming, there will be frequent shivering and chills, dull, heavy, throbbing pain, and a feeling of numbness in the loin, and the fever cools. Sometimes the abscess bursts inside, and the matter comes away with the urine; this may be known by examining the water, and you will see a thick stuff, which settles down to the bottom of the pot by itself; but if it mixes up with the water, you may conclude that it is not matter from an abscess, but only a sediment caused by inflammation of the kidneys or bladder. When the patient is about to get better, without an abscess, these will be the symptoms : the pain and fever abate, the skin all over the body becomes moist, the sickness and puking are checked, the water flows freely, is muddy, or mixed with slime, called mucus. An abscess in the kidneys is always to be avoided, if possible.

Treatment.—Bleed immediately, and then cup the loins. When the cups are removed, put a large, soft, warm poultice to the loins, and purge out the bowels with this ;

12 grains of calomel, or blue pill,

40 grains comp. extract colocynth,

made into six pills ; give one pill every hour, until the bowels are well opened—and if they do not purge well, give a dose of castor-oil two hours after the last pill. About evening, give two or three injections of this (warm) ;

1 quart of flaxseed tea,

½ wineglass of laudanum, mixed.

11

The patient must drink freely of flaxseed-tea, say a cupful, having in it one grain of Dover's powder, every two or three hours, day and night. You must also surround the patient's body with hot bricks, wrapped in flannels which have been wet with vinegar and water, and put under the bed-covering. After you have continued this treatment from twelve to twenty-four hours, if the pain in the loins is not relieved, and the urine does not flow freely, you must put a blister over the place which was cupped, and when the blister has been on four or five hours, take it off, and put on the place a large warm mustard-poultice (see page 68), and put on another when this gets hard. Keep the bowels open from day to day with mild purges, as Epsom salts, &c. After the inflammation and severe pain in the loin have been subdued, there is apt to be a soreness in the loin, in one or both sides. When this is the case, give this:—

    25 grains of uva ursi,
     3 grains Dover's powder,

made into one powder. Give a powder every three or four hours during the day; give very light food for nourishment.

INFLAMMATION OF THE BLADDER.

Symptoms.— A severe burning, shooting, or throbbing pain over the privates, which sometimes shoots down to the testicles, fundament, and thighs. The place near the fundament feels sore when you touch it, and that over the privates more painful when you press on it.   The patient tries often to pass water, and strains, without being able to pass but a very small quantity, and that deep red and often bloody. Sometimes the water comes away constantly, in drops. Very often, sick stomach and puking; oppression of the chest; bowels costive, and sometimes a straining; pulse quick, hard, and full; great thirst, hot and dry skin, restlessness and melancholy. These symptoms vary at times, according as one or another part of the bladder is principally inflamed. This disease generally lasts for about six or seven days, and ends in mortification of the bladder, or the patient gets better; and sometimes, but rarely, matter is found in the bladder. When mortification is about to take place, the pain ceases suddenly, the hands and feet become cold, a clammy sweat comes over the body, the patient becomes very weak, his face very pale, his mind somewhat composed, pulse weak and quick, &c.

When the patient is about to get better, the pain ceases or lessens; a warm sweat comes over the whole body; the water comes away plentifully, and with no pain, but looks muddy; and he can bear pressure over the privates.

Treatment.—Bleed immediately until the pulse is reduced, and put leeches about the fundament and over the privates, and as soon as the leeches come away, put warm poultices over the leech-bites. Give a dose of castor oil, and two or three injections of flaxseed-tea, until the bowels have been well emptied. Then give an anodyne clyster (see page 70). Next, sweat the patient with bricks, in the manner directed in page 122; and let him use, as a drink, the mixture of flaxseed-tea, with Dover's powder, recommended in the same page. If there is now a stoppage of water, you must introduce a silver catheter: get directions from a physician. Let the patient sit down in a tub of warm water several times during the day. If the disease still remains obstinate, use this :—

  2 grains of calomel, or 3 of blue pill,
  1 grain of opium, or 4 of Dover's powder,
made into one powder. Give a powder every four hours until the patient is relieved. Last of all, when these remedies fail, put a blister over the privates, and do after as recommended for the kidneys, page 121.

———

CHRONIC INFLAMMATION OF THE BLADDER.

THIS disease sometimes arises from the same cause which produces the disease just described, or it may remain as a consequence of it.

Symptoms.—A feeling of weight and tenderness near the fundament; a heat or burning, and slight shooting pains, over the privates; a desire to pass water continually, and frequent spasm of the bladder and water-passage. The water is filled with a thick and sometimes ropy slime or mucus.

Weakness, slow fever, and thirst. The digestion, too, is generally bad; sometimes sickness and puking; bowels costive, skin harsh and dry, tongue covered with a white or brown fur. Some other symptoms appear, more or less numerous, according to the severity of the case.

Treatment.—If the pulse is full and active, and much pain about the privates, bleed moderately; then cup the loins, and put leeches now and then about the fundament. Keep the bowels constantly loose by giving a dose of castor-oil or magnesia every now and then.—(See pages 32 and 33.) If the disease remains obstinate, rub the loins with tartar-emetic ointment. The patient must drink constantly of flaxseed-tea, or slippery-elm tea, made by pouring a pint of boiling water on a teaspoonful of the elm-bark. He may take one of these pills every night and morning also:—

    15 grains of uva ursi,
    $\frac{1}{2}$ grain of the extract of hyosciamus,

made into one pill. If these remedies do not succeed (as the disease is sometimes very obstinate), try the balsam-Copaiva capsules. Give one three times a day. Remember, the patient must take only the simplest food, and no spirituous liquors, but use such drinks as flaxseed-tea, barley-water, &c.; must not ride on horseback, or take hard exercise. Sometimes two or three grains of super-carbonate of soda, mixed with the drinks, gives relief.

INFLAMMATION OF THE WOMB.

This generally occurs in females just after child-birth.

Symptoms.—A fixed, dull, aching, or shooting pain between the hips, with a feeling of weight or bearing down near the fundament, generally increased by motion, or when pressed upon. Urine stopped, or passed with much pain and difficulty. The pain may be more or less severe, and differently located, according to the part of the womb to which the inflammation is principally confined. Sometimes the pains are in paroxysms, like after-pains, but may be distinguished from them with little difficulty. Frequently the after-discharge is stopped, but not always; severe headache, and delirium toward evening; sick stomach, and puking now and then. Pulse full, strong, and hard—sometimes small, quick, and contracted; bowels generally slow; urine small in quantity, of a deep-red color, and passed with pain and difficulty. This disease is apt to end in suppuration or mortification of the womb if the patient does not get better in four or five days, though these results are not very common. These are the symptoms when the womb alone is inflamed; but when it involves the peritoneum, it is called *puerperal fever*, and these are the

Symptoms.—The pulse becomes quicker, the lower part of the stomach swells and becomes very tender; great weakness; the patient lies on her back, with the knees and shoulders raised; tongue dry and covered with a brown coat, and sometimes looseness of the bowels, particularly toward the termination of the disease. When the patient is about to get better, the pain and tenderness of the womb decrease; the pulse becomes soft and slower, the tongue clean and moist, the skin soft and moist; the urine flows more freely, and the other symptoms become better. When mortification (which seldom occurs) is about to take place, you will notice the usual symptoms of mortification, which I have described.

Suppuration, or the formation of matter in the womb, is very dangerous, particularly if the matter is discharged in the cavity of the belly. When it is about to happen, you will notice these symptoms: slight chills and heat passing irregularly over the body; a weight in the womb, and a lessening of the pain after five or six days; great weakness; dry, red tongue; a flush in one or both cheeks; cool sweats in different parts of the body, and the discharge from the privates increased and offensive.

Treatment.—Bleed immediately, and if the pulse does not become soft and the pain abate, bleed again, and again, until they do. Put leeches, if they can be had, over the privates and about the privates, and as soon as the leeches come off, put warm poultices to the leech-bites, apply them from time to time as fast as they get hard. Then give this: 8 or 10 grains of calomel, and four hours afterward a dose of Epsom salts.—(See table.) Put blisters to the inner part of the thighs, high up, and give clysters of warm flaxseed-tea, or warm milk and water, frequently. When the bowels have

11*

been well purged out with the calomel and the salts, give this :—

          36 grains of Dover's powder,
          12 grains of Calomel,

made into six powders. Give one powder every three or four hours during the day. The patient must drink freely of flaxseed-tea. Two grains of James' powder, mixed with two grains of saltpetre (powdered), every night and morning, will do much good when there is not much irritability of the stomach. If these remedies do no good, give this :—

          1 grain of powdered opium,
          2 grains of calomel,

made into one powder, and given every three hours ; and put a large blister over the womb, above the privates.

————

CHRONIC INFLAMMATION OF THE WOMB.

THIS disease is very common, and very apt to be mistaken or neglected. The inflammation in most cases is seated principally in the neck and mouth of the womb.

Symptoms.—Sometimes only a heat low down in the womb, or dull, shooting pains, which go and come. Sometimes a weight and pain in the upper parts of the privates. The patient generally has the whites, which often looks like matter. This disease may last for many years, and at last cause an incurable disease of the womb. Females, therefore, should never neglect attending to the whites.

Treatment.—The treatment in this disease does not differ materially from that of inflammation of the womb, only you need not give such large doses. When you have bled, the necessity for which must be determined by the pulse, and purged out the bowels, &c., if the whites still remain, see the directions for the whites, and follow them.

If the disease is obstinate, you may put blisters, about the size of your hand, to the back, just above the fundament, and if there is not much inflammation, you may give a few drops of balsam copaiva twice or three times a day.

PLEURISY.

Symptoms.—A severe sticking pain in the chest, on one side or the other, which is increased when the patient draws a deep breath, or coughs. Breathing short and quick. Short and dry cough, with a colorless spittle. Sometimes there is blood in the spittle, and then you may know that the lungs are inflamed also. Hot and dry skin; urine small in quantity and deep red; tongue covered with a thick white fur; face flushed, pulse very hard, full and quick. The patient tries to keep his ribs from moving, and uses the muscles of his belly to breathe with. Notice this—these symptoms do not always appear as there is sometimes very little pain and cough, and yet much inflammation.

Treatment.—Bleed from a large orifice, until the pain is lessened, and the pulse falls, and if it rise again, you must bleed again, and again, with judgment, until it is removed. Put a good blister over the place where the pain is, and give this :—

　　12 grains of calomel,
　　12 grains of Dover's powder,

made into two or three powders, and give one every two or three hours, until they operate; four or five hours afterward, give a·moderate dose of castor-oil, or Epsom salts. The patient must drink, every two or three hours during the day, some of the senega, or senpentaria.—(See page 37.) Or, if the skin is not very dry, flaxseed tea. If you find the skin obstinately dry, put about two grains of the antimonial powder or six drops of the antimonial wine, or six grains of salt-petre, to every cup of the snake-root, which must be given hot. Keep the bowels open from day to day, with one or two moderate doses of some mild purge, or the calomel and Dover's powder as directed. You will find the life-everlasting tea, an excellent thing to use as a sweat, particularly if you have not the snake-root. This is not a dangerous disease in strong healthy persons, but sometimes in weak constitutions, it is dangerous, as it may bring on consumption. The bad symptoms are these :—Bloody spittle, a wheezing in the throat, loose bowels, convulsions, while the patient is constantly trying to sit up. When these symptoms appear, you must treat it like the following disease.

PERIPNEUMONY, OR INFLAMMATION OF THE LUNGS.

In this disease, the substance of the lungs is principally inflamed, and these are the

Symptoms.—Difficulty of breathing when the patient is lying down; dull pain in the chest, generally about the breast bone; sometimes about the pit of the stomach, and sometimes about the shoulder-blade. Cough, and spitting up a quantity of clear glairy stuff, sometimes mixed with blood. Pulse quick, full, and laboring, but not generally hard, weak and irregular when the disease is advanced. When the disease is very violent, and the inflamed portion of the lungs is about to be disorganized, or water to form on the lungs, you will observe these symptoms :—The spittle white, yellowish, or greenish, with bubbles in it, and sticks close to the vessel. Sometimes, however, the disease becomes dangerous, and a considerable portion of the lungs disorganized, without any conspicuous symptoms.

Treatment.—As this disease is nearly allied to pleurisy, the treatment is not materially different. It is not necessary to take so much blood, and, in fact, blood, in many cases, must be taken with much caution, as when the pulse is weak, instead of bleeding, give this : a wineglassful of the root of poligala, or senega; pour a pint of boiling water on this, and let it boil about half an hour. Then put in one grain of tartar emetic, and give a wineglassful of the mixture, warm, every hour. As a general rule, keep the bowels open by giving this :—

    2 grains of calomel,
    1 grain of hippo, or antimonial powder,

every two hours during the day, and four or five hours after the last dose, give a dose of castor-oil or Epsom salts.—(See *Table.*) The patient may drink freely, from time to time, of flaxseed tea, and if the pain in the chest is obstinate, put a blister between the shoulders, and to the calves of the legs, if necessary. Lastly, if the patient begins to sink, give this :—

    1 grain of camphor,
    1 grain of powdered opium,

rubbed up with a little white sugar, and taken every hour, and to produce perspiration, when the skin is obstinately dry.

    1 grain of tartar emetic,
    4 grains of saltpetre (powdered),

made into eight powders. Give one powder every hour.

BILIOUS PLEURISY.

This disease is a modification of pneumonia, or inflammation of the lungs.

Symptoms.—White tongue, with a yellowish streak along the middle, at the commencement of the disease; afterward, dark, brown, and dry. Pulse generally small and quick, and somewhat tight, like a cord. Frequently, the patient feels, when the disease is coming on, considerable pain in the back and legs; sometimes a fulness and tightness in the right side; and sometimes the bowels are loose, just before the fever comes on. The skin and the whites of the eyes generally tinged with bile; face flushed and yellowish. Sharp pain in the forehead. Pain in the chest, sometimes very severe and burning, but more commonly dull, with weight and oppression in the breast. Sometimes the fever lasts for several days before the pain in the breast comes on. The patient does not spit much, and what he spits is yellowish and frothy, and marked frequently with streaks of blood. The fever generally rises in the evening, and cools in the morning. There is generally puking of bilious matter, but sometimes what comes up, has no bile in it, but only the mucus, and contents of the stomach. Urine always yellow and bilious. When the patient is about to get better, you will see a gentle perspiration, the cough will become less troublesome, and the pain and oppression of the chest will abate; the urine flow more freely, and have a sediment in it; and he will spit up a quantity of thick yellowish matter.

But if what he spits up becomes dark, or red and watery, the cough becomes dry, the pain and oppression spread through the whole chest, with a feeling of suffocation, the face and lips blue, the pulse soft, laboring, and irregular, if the inside of the body feels cold, while the outside is still very warm, and other bad symptoms appear, the patient is in great danger. This, however, is a very treacherous disease, and sometimes the patient may get better, when the worst symptoms appear, and die, when very few bad symptoms are seen.

Treatment.—Bleed immediately, but be careful to keep your finger on the pulse, while the blood is running. If you find the pulse rise, let the blood run until it falls again; then tie up the arm. Next give an emetic of hippo (see page 46), and when the patient has thrown up once or twice, so as to

remove everything in his stomach, put a large blister between
his shoulders, which must be dressed with warm poultices,
when it comes off, for a day or two, and give this;

     12 grains of calomel,
     8 grains of antimonial powder,
     4 grains of camphor,

rubbed up, and made into six powders. Give one powder
every hour, until they produce two or three good large bilious passages; then, four or five hours after the last powder,
give a dose of castor-oil. Remember, both in this disease and
peripneumony, all the bleeding must be done in the first
twenty-four hours, for afterward bleeding is dangerous unless
practised with great caution and judgment. With regard to
the rest of the treatment in this disease, follow the directions
for peripneumony. After the inflammation and pain in the
chest have been relieved in a measure, give the senega and
tartar emetic, as directed for peripneumony (see page 128).
Some physicians speak highly of the muriate and carbonate
of ammonia, in this and peripneumony, but, as I have never
used them much, I can not recommend them. You may
give an emetic of hippo, every now and then, during this disease (but not in peripneumony), if the pain in the chest is
obstinate, and the skin is very dry and hot.

INFLAMMATION OF THE LARYNX.

This disease is apt to be mistaken for croup, but by attention to the symptoms, you will distinguish it. Soreness in
the throat, uneasiness in swallowing, and tenderness when
the throat is pressed upon. The voice changed to a thick,
hoarse whisper, and when the breath is drawn in, it sounds
hoarse, dull, and hollow, as if passing through a narrow opening. If you look into the throat, you will find it pale, red,
swollen, and dropsical. The patient does not spit much, but
what he spits is ropy. Pulse generally quick, small, and
tight; tongue white, with red points and covered with a layer of clear mucus, &c. The patient is unable to cough out.
This is a dangerous disease and requires the most prompt
treatment.

Treatment.—Bleed immediately until the patient faints; then put several leeches to the throat, and a good-sized blister to the back of the neck. When the leeches drop off, apply warm soft poultices to the leech-bites, and then give an emetic of tartar emetic (see page 46). When the patient has puked twice, or three times, let him remain quiet for an hour, with his feet in warm water and mustard. Then give this, if a child five or six years old, half if younger;

     5 grains of calomel,
     5 grains of jalap, or rhubarb,

rubbed up and made into one powder. If it does not purge in three hours, give another powder of the same, and four or five hours afterward, a dose of castor-oil, or Epsom salts. When this disease will not yield to this treatment, send for a physician, and let him perform the operation of tracheotomy. But remember, you have no time to lose.

ACUTE BRONCHITIS.

Symptoms.—Not much pain, but great oppression and tightness in the breast, severe pain in the forehead, which is much increased by coughing; a wheezing and rattling sound, when the patient breathes, uneasiness when lying down, some fever, face pale, and a quantity of clear, frothy mucus comes up every now and then from the chest.

Treatment.—Bleed cautiously, particularly if the patient is weak or old. Keep the bowels open with injections and mild cathartics, as castor-oil and Epsom salts. Give an emetic every now and then, of hippo, antimonial wine, or squills. (See pages 46 and 47.) This will also be found a good mixture every now and then; decoction of senega (see page 37). A half pint of this to a wineglassful of the oxymel of squills, mixed together. Give a tablespoonful of this mixture every two hours, to a grown person. If the patient becomes very weak, stimulate with camphor.—(See page 14.) Lastly, put blisters over the chest, and as soon as they make the place red, take them off, and put on warm poultices.

PERICARDITIS, OR INFLAMMATION OF THE BAG WHICH SURROUNDS THE HEART.

Symptoms.—Sudden, severe, cutting pains in the middle of the chest, reaching sometimes to the pit of the stomach, or to the back, between the shoulders; difficulty of breathing, palpitation of the heart, and a feeling of weight and tightness in the left side of the chest, under the breast-bone. Irregular pulse; the patient prefers sitting up to lying down; and generally sits leaning forward, with his head resting on a chair. If he moves from this posture, it causes him the most severe, sharp pains in his chest. Sometimes sudden feelings, as if he was going to faint, a short, dry cough, and oppression of the chest. The pulse generally irregular, and stops every now and then, or very weak. Several other symptoms appear and these symptoms vary, more or less, according to circumstances. There is no disease, which differs more in its symptoms than this at different times.

Treatment.—Bleed with judgment, the quantity of blood to be taken to depend upon the state of the pulse, and the strength of the patient. Put large blisters between the shoulders, and leeches to the chest, and then warm poultices over the leech-bites. Keep the bowels open with calomel and opium, in this way;

> 12 grains of calomel,
> 4 grains of opium,

made into four powders. Give one powder every three hours. If the disease is obstinate, go on with this until you salivate. In other respects, treat the disease according to the directions given for peripneumony.

CHRONIC PERICARDITIS.

THIS form of this disease is much more common than the acute, and its symptoms are similar, but not so severe. The feet and legs of persons laboring under this disease, are apt to be puffy at times, and sometimes the face, particularly under the eyes. And patients are timid, weak-minded, and easily alarmed, and have a mean, pusillanimous look.

Treatment.—The treatment, also, does not differ materially from that of the acute, only it need not be so severe. Calomel, combined with squills, is good in this manner:—

        12 grains of calomel,
        3 grains of powdered squills,

rubbed up, and made into six powders ; give one powder every two hours, and continue this treatment for some time, together with blisters kept regularly to the back, between the shoulders. To keep the bowels regularly open, in this and in the acute form, give this ;—

        12 grains of calomel,
        2 teaspoonfuls of cream of tartar,

rubbed well together, and made into six powders ; give one powder every two or three hours during the day.

ACUTE RHEUMATISM.

Symptoms.—The symptoms which precede an attack of this disease, do not differ materially from those of other diseases arising from colds. It generally comes on with pain in several joints or parts of the body, sometimes with fever. Some of these parts now become swollen, red, and very painful ; the pain is of a gnawing, tearing kind, generally increased when the patient is warm in bed. The pulse is now generally full, strong, and quick, skin hot and dry ; tongue covered with a white fur, which afterward becomes brown. The bowels are costive, great thirst, &c.

Treatment.—Bleed with care and judgment ; next purge out the bowels with this :—

        12 grains of calomel,
        12 grains of Dover's powder.

rubbed up, and made into two powders ; give one three hours after the other, and four or five hours after the last powder, give a dose of Epsom salts, or rhubarb. (See pages 32 and 33.) The bowels must be kept constantly open with this :—

        2 tablespoonfuls of Epsom salts,
        1 grain of tartar emetic,

dissolved in a half pint of water ; give a tablespoonful every
12

hour, from day to day, and every night and morning, one of those powders :—

    3 grains of calomel,
    3 grains of Dover's powder, or 1 grain of powdered
        opium.

An emetic of hippo, or antimonial wine, every now and then, will be found very beneficial. Lastly, if after all this treatment, the disease remains obstinate, give this :—

    2 grains of calomel,
    1 grain of powdered opium,

made into one powder; to be taken every three or four hours, until the gums are a little sore, then stop, and three or four hours afterward, give a moderate dose of castor-oil, or Epsom salts.

BILIOUS RHEUMATISM.

This is common in swampy and unhealthy parts of the country.

Symptoms.—Pain in the head, eyes yellowish, sick stomach and puking sometimes; a thick layer of brown fur on the tongue; the stuff which comes from the stomach full of bile, and other symptoms of rheumatism. The treatment of this form does not differ materially from the acute; it requires, in some cases, to be treated like bilious intermitting fever.

CHRONIC RHEUMATISM.

The symptoms which characterize this disease are sufficiently conspicuous not to require a particular description.

Treatment.—Look to the state of the bowels. If they are bound, give every night, or every other night, five or six grains of blue pill, and the next morning give a dose of the compound tincture of rhubarb (a wineglassful). If the patient is weak and relaxed, sulphate of quinine, in this proportion, is useful:—

    6 grains sulphate quinine,
    1 drop of sulphuric acid, or 3 drops of the elixir of
        vitriol, in a half-pint of water.

Take a wineglassful three or four times a day. This also is good in weak habits, but if the patient is strong and healthy, and it is apt to do harm, one tablespoonful ammoniated tincture of guiacum to a half-pint of water: give a tablespoonful four times a day. If the disease is obstinate, touch the gums slightly with calomel and opium. A great number of remedies have been recommended, as turpentine, sulphate of zinc, savin, colchicum, stramonium, hyosciamus, &c. You may try these in small doses, if the others fail. Apply to a physician for the dose.

Sometimes great benefit is derived from warm baths at night, and winding flannel bandages tight around the afflicted joints. If all these means fail, you must carry the patient, if possible, to the warm springs of North Carolina. I have seen some wonderful cures of this disease, in the last stage, effected by bathing constantly from day to day in the warm bath of these springs.

INFLAMMATION OF THE EYES FROM COLD.

Symptoms.—The patient feels a pain in the eyes, can not bear the light, and has a constant feeling of sand in his eyes. Great flow of tears, and sometimes matter runs, instead of tears. Very little headache, and not much fever.

Treatment.—If the pulse is full and high, bleed moderately, and cup the back of the neck; then purge out the bowels with this:—

    8 grains of calomel,
    20 grains of jalap,

made into one powder. Five or six hours after this, give a good dose of Epsom or Glauber salts. The bowels must be kept constantly loose with purgatives, as Epsom salts, &c. Wash the eyes with warm milk and water, or elder-blossom tea. If the disease is obstinate, put blisters to the back of the neck ; and if after the inflammation is subdued, the eyes still remain red, use this :—

    4 grains of the nitrate of silver,

in a wineglass of rain-water. Drop a drop or two of this, with a feather, into the eye, three or four times a day. If the patient remains feverish, and the eyes painful and irritable, give this :—

    1 grain of calomel,
    18 grains of Dover's powder,

made into six powders ; give one powder every three or four hours in the day. This disease sometimes is very obstinate, and defies treatment. In such cases, put a seton back of the neck, and keep it there.

———   .

RHEUMATIC INFLAMMATION OF THE EYES.

Symptoms.—Severe pain around the eyeballs, which extends to the temples, lower jaw, and inside of the ear. The pain increases at night ; the whites of the eyes of a yellowish red ; flow of tears—at first not great, afterward copious. Sometimes ulcers form on the ball of the eye, and matter inside.

Symptoms.—If the pulse is high, bleed moderately, and give an emetic of tartar emetic or antimonial wine.—(See page 46.) Next purge out the bowels in the manner recommended for inflammation of the eyes from cold, and use the same treatment. After the bowels have been well purged out, you may give this :—

    6 grains of calomel,
    6 grains of antimonial powder,
    1 grain of powdered opium,

made into six powders ; give one powder every two hours, and continue them for some time. Use this also :—

    4 grains of sulphate of morphine ;

pour on it a wineglassful of boiling water. Drop this into the eye several times a day with a feather.

PURULENT INFLAMMATION OF THE EYES, CALLED PURULENT OPHTHALMIA.

Symptoms.—Severe shooting pains through the eye; eyelids soon swell enormously. A quantity of matter comes away in large drops from under the eyelids. Pain in the head very severe, high fever, increasing toward evening. About the third or fourth day, the severe symptoms begin to abate, or else the patient loses his sight.

Treatment.—In severe cases bleed immediately, and if the pain and inflammation do not abate, bleed again and again, remembering that all the bleeding must be confined to the first twenty-hours. Put several leeches around the eye; purge out the bowels well, and follow the directions for rheumatic inflammation of the eyes. The treatment must depend upon the severity of the symptoms.

SCROFULOUS INFLAMMATION OF THE EYES.

This disease occurs more frequently in children than in grown persons.

Symptoms.—Great discharge from the eyes during sleep, which causes the eyelids to stick together; eyes very sensible to the light; not much pain; colored part of the eye red. Sometimes little spots form on the eyeball, which, after a while, break and form ulcers, which extend to the inside of the eye, and let out the humors.

Treatment.—This disease does not require such active treatment as the other forms just described; but you must purge out the bowels, and keep them open with calomel and jalap, or rhubarb. Follow the general directions for the other forms. With regard to the particular treatment, I must refer you to a physician. Concerning the other diseases of the eye, as syphilitic and strumous iritis, amaurosis, &c., I will not attempt to give any directions, as they will require the management of physicians.

12*

PUKING BLOOD.

PUT a large mustard-plaster over the stomach (see page 68); put the feet into a warm pediluvium (see page 68); give clysters (see page 70); give purges of rhubarb or jalap (see pages 32 and 33), until the bowels are well emptied, particularly if the patient is a female, as it frequently arises from a stoppage of the monthly discharge. Keep the patient as quiet as possible, and give the lightest nourishment. If these do no good, give emetics of hippo.

———

BLEEDING FROM THE WOMB.

I WOULD have you understand that I am not speaking of bleeding from the womb after child-birth, but of it as it occurs in females who are not in a family way; and, at the same time, remember, I do not mean a great increase of the monthly discharge, but blood which clots, and which you know is not the case with the monthly courses, for they never clot. Remember this.

Symptoms which precede an attack.—Frequent desire to make water, heaviness in the head, and ringing noise in the ears; a feeling of weight in the feet; pain and fullness in the loins and between the hips; a feeling of fullness and bearing down in the womb; pulse sometimes small, weak, and quick, or full, bounding, or wavering; chills, with flushes of heat every now and then. These symptoms, however, do not always precede an attack, for frequently the blood gushes away suddenly, and runs for two, three, or four hours, and stops. But it frequently also continues to run for four or five days, or as many weeks, and stops by degrees.

Treatment.—If the pulse is quick and tight, like a cord, bleed moderately, and make the patient lie as still and quiet as possible. Then give this:—

      12 grains of sugar of lead,
       6 grains of hippo,

rubbed up, and made up into six powders; give one of these

powders every hour, or even half hour, until the bleeding is checked. If the patient is of a weak constitution, or much weakened from the bleeding, add a grain of camphor to each of the powders, well rubbed up. Put cloths wet with cold water over the womb and to the privates; and if the bleeding is obstinate, you must push a piece of soft lint, wet with vinegar and water, into the privates. Five or six grains of Dover's powders at night, also, will be found useful.

PHLEGMASIA DOLENS.

This disease generally occurs from five to nine days after child-birth.

Symptoms.—Chills and ague, followed by pain and stiffness in the groin of one side; then a swelling of the leg, which soon extends over the whole limb—the feet being sometimes swelled to an enormous size, and very painful.

Treatment.—Bleed at the commencement of the disease, and put leeches to the groin of the affected side, and even down the leg. The bleeding from the arm must be repeated from time to time, until the inflammatory symptoms are reduced. Next purge out the bowels well with magnesia and Epsom salts (see page 32), and give this:—

20 grains of Dover's powder,
50 grains of saltpetre,
6 grains of calomel,

made into twelve powders. Give one every two hours during the day and night. Apply flannels wrung out in hot water constantly to the leech-bites, and if these do not give relief, apply warm anodyne poultices.—(See page 68.) As a general rule, do not use warm poultices in the early part of the disease; but when the pain and swelling are somewhat relieved, then they may be used. After the application of these, much benefit may be derived from rubbing the affected limb with whiskey, and bandaging it from the toes to the hips with bandages which have been wetted with strong salt and water and dried. When the patient is recovering, she must take gentle exercise in walking, and if very weak, use some of the tonics.—(See from page 64 to 67.)

APOPLEXY.

THE symptoms which generally precede an attack of this disease are giddiness, a dull and deep-seated pain, or a feeling of weight in the head, which the patient feels particularly when he stoops or turns his head suddenly round; ringing in the ears; dimness of sight, sparks and flashes of light before the eyes, drowsiness, heavy sleep, and many other symptoms which indicate some disorder about the brain. These symptoms may last for weeks, months, or a longer period, or only for a few hours before the fit comes on. Sometimes the fit comes on suddenly, the patient being deprived of motion, and falling down in a kind of stupor, like a deep sleep. This last form of the attack is very dangerous, and requires the most prompt treatment. Sometimes, again, the patient feels a sudden, deep-seated pain in the head; he is seized with a trembling of his hands and feet, confusion of mind, giddiness in the head, sickness and puking, when he soon sinks down, unable to move. Sometimes he soon recovers from this state and can walk about and converse, still feeling a giddiness and other unpleasant sensations in his head; but in a few hours the bad symptoms return, the head becomes more and more oppressed, and the patient sinks down, as if in a deep sleep. If you feel the pulse now, you will find it weak, the breathing is weak, sometimes scarcely perceptible; soon, however, the breathing becomes stronger, and has a sound like snoring; the pulse becomes regular, full, and frequently hard.

Treatment.—Lay the patient down, with his head slightly raised, then open the vein of the arm and let the blood flow; shave the head, and apply cold wet cloths to the scalp. Put mustard-plasters to the legs and feet (see page 68). Cup the temples and back of the neck. If the attack is a very severe one, bleed from the jugular vein or temporal artery. The blood must run until the pulse is evidently affected, and if it rises in an hour or so, you must bleed again and again, if necessary. If you can get medicine down the throat, give this:

A large wineglassful of castor-oil,
A teaspoonful of spirits of turpentine.

Or this:—

15 grains of calomel,
15 grains of jalap,

at one dose, for a grown person; or any active purge which you can get quickly.—(See *Cathartics.*) 'Give injections freely, 30 or 40 grains of aloes, to a pint of water. In severe cases, this :—

    10 grains of tartar emetic,

    To a pint of warm water, with a little soap in it.

As a general rule, emetics are dangerous in this disease, but if the patient has just eaten a hearty meal, or his stomach is loaded with irritating matter, give an emetic immediately. The sulphate of zinc is good—from 15 to 20 grains dissolved in water. Lastly, if you can not get medicine down the throat, take 3 drops of croton-oil, mix it with a little water, and pour it in the mouth. It would be as well, also, to put several mustard plasters over different parts of the body, so as to induce a determination of blood from the head, when the patient has been relieved, and to prevent the rush of blood again to the head.

CONVULSIONS, OR FITS IN INFANTS.

THESE may be produced by various causes, as worms, indigestible food, any irritating substances in the stomach or bowels, blows, or falls on the head, and teething.

Symptoms.—It is difficult to give the exact symptoms of convulsions, but you may know them by these. A peculiar jerking of the muscles of the body and limbs, jaws clenched, eyes squinting, &c. Sometimes the muscles of the back are permanently contracted, so as to bend the body backward, and there may be foam issuing from the closed lips.

Treatment.—The treatment must depend principally upon the cause which produces the fits. If from indigestible food, or you have reason to suppose so, give an emetic of hippo immediately (see page 46), and if the pulse is full and hard, bleed from the arm, in severe cases, from the jugular vein. Next purge out the bowels with castor-oil and turpentine— a tablespoonful of the oil, to ten drops of turpentine, for a child three or four years old, half for one younger. Put the child into a warm bath up to the hips, and pour cold water over the head and shoulders. But if you find the face become pale, or the pulse sink, stop with the cold water; this may be done from the very first. If the fits are obstinate, put blisters behind the ears, and to the temples, or even between the shoulders, and to the calves of the legs, and you may rub the chest and body with spirits of camphor, or dry mustard, or anything irritating. If the fits are produced by worms, follow the directions for worms. As a general rule, treat all cases of convulsions in the way I have described, unless the pulse is very low, or the child very weak from illness; then you must depend principally upon blisters and small doses of opium, say one grain of powdered opium, to three grains of calomel, made into six powders; give one powder every half hour, until the fits cease, or instead of the opium, four grains of Dover's powder, in the same way. A dose of calomel every now and then, will be useful (see page 31), and I have sometimes relieved fits, when obstinate, with this:—

        A teaspoonful of laudanum,
        2 grains of tartar emetic,

made into two doses; give one a half hour after the other. It is rather a dangerous remedy, though a good one.

CONVULSIONS, OR FITS FROM TEETHING.

This form of convulsions is somewhat peculiar in its symptoms, and requires to be noticed very particularly, though not very dangerous, if taken in time.

Symptoms.—A hurried breathing, with a sound as if there was a quantity of mucus in the wind-pipe, when the child awakes from sleep. The face becomes pale, shrivelled, and anxious, the nose pinched, and the child frowns almost constantly, and when it is put to the breast, seizes it, but immediately jerks away again. The symptoms may last a longer or a shorter time, according to circumstances, when you will observe the thumbs pressed upon the palms of the hand, and the wrists and ankle joints drawn inward, and the head oftentimes thrown backward. The noise in breathing now is like croup, and the child sobs, but does not cry, during the fits. After a while convulsive movements of parts of the whole

body generally, comes on.   The bowels are generally bound,
Not much fever generally.   These symptoms may continue
for some time.

Treatment.—If the gums are swollen, cut them down to
the tooth which is coming; in other respects, the treatment
does not differ from the first variety.

CONVULSIONS OF PREGNANT WOMEN—AND DURING AND AFTER CHILD-BIRTH, CALLED PUERPERAL CONVULSIONS.

Symptoms.—Just before the fit the following symptoms appear.   Giddiness, ringing in the ears, blindness every now
and then, a feeling of fullness, weight, tightness, and a deep-
seated pain in the head.   The blood-vessels of the head are
generally full, and sometimes there is a severe dull pain in
the stomach, and weakness of the legs.   These symptoms
may continue for some time, when suddenly the fits come on
with a severe jerking of the muscles of the face and body.
During the fits, the face is flushed, and the blood settles in it,
the tongue thrust out between the teeth, breathing quick, a
sputtering of the lips; and when the fit is about to terminate,
a quantity of frothy stuff comes from the mouth.

Treatment.—The treatment of this disease does not differ
essentially from that of apoplexy.—(See pages 140 and 141.)
and must be regulated according to its violence.   As a general rule, bleed immediately, and if you can get anything
down the throat, give this:—

  10 grains of calomel,
  10 grains of jalap,
   6 grains of powdered aloes,

rubbed together, and made into one powder; to be taken at
one dose.   Give clysters (see page 70), until the bowels are
well emptied.   Put mustard plasters to the ankles and calves
of the legs (see page 68), and cold cloths, or even ice, to the
head.   In severe cases, shave the head, put pounded ice in a
bladder, and cup the temples and back of the neck.   If the
case is severe, and the woman is near her time, try and deliver

her immediately. If the womb will not contract (see directions for *forcing delivery*) pass a probe up the vagina, and break the bag of waters. This form of puerperal convulsions which I have just described, is very violent and dangerous; but there is another form of the same disease, called hysteric convulsions, which are not so dangerous, in which the determination of blood to the head is by no means as great, and consequently do not require such severe and active treatment.

Symptoms.—The face is not as much flushed, as in the other variety, and sometimes somewhat pale; no frothing at the mouth. The large muscles jerk violently, and those of the back are contracted, so that the head and heels are bent backward, while the breast and belly are bent forward like a bow. The patient also may even converse after the fit, though she will be very stupid, and is apt to look wildly about the room for a moment or so, and then hide her head, as if ashamed.

Treatment.—In this form, it will generally be necessary to take only a pint, or a pint and a half of blood, unless the pulse is full and hard, or you see symptoms of a rush of blood to the head, as flushed face, or blood settling in the face; then take more blood, until these symptoms are removed. Next, empty the bowels with clysters.—(See page 70.) Put mustard plasters to the legs and ankles. If the fits return, give a full dose of laudanum (see page 29), and give an anodyne clyster of asafœtida (see page 70).

TETANUS, OR SPASMS,

MAY be caused by poisonous substances, some of the narcotic poisons, unwholesome food, exposure to cold or damp when the body is heated; but most frequently from wounds about tendinous parts, as the foot and hand. It occurs, also, in infants, just after birth, and is commonly called locked-jaw. It is a very dangerous disease, particularly in infants, and when it arises from wounds. You must be careful not to confound this disease with convulsions; for in convulsions, the mind is always affected, and the patient knows nothing, or very little of

what is going on around him ; Whereas, in tetanus, the patient never loses his mind, and not even his appetite.

Symptoms.—When the disease is coming on, the patient
will feel slight spasms, or cramps about the throat; he does
not swallow as well as usual, and his voice is somewhat
changed. About this time, also, he has an uneasy feeling
about the heart, and soon afterward he feels a stiffness in his
neck, and about his shoulders. The jaws now begin to be
stiff, but not so much as to prevent the patient from opening
his mouth. This stiffness increases, however, until the jaws
are firmly locked together. You will observe now, that the
patient's head is drawn back, and he feels sudden and painful
jerks near the pit of the stomach. He swallows with difficulty
and pain. The pain and jerking at the pit of the stomach,
now return about every quarter of an hour, and become very
violent ; the head is drawn back powerfully, and almost every
muscle of the body is stiff and hard. These spasms last only
for a few minutes, when all the muscles, except those of the
jaws, become relaxed, or loose, when the spasms come on
again. As the disease advances, the spasms become more
severe, and all the symptoms are aggravated, &c.

Treatment.—If the disease has been produced by a cut, or
wound of any kind, lay the place open with a sharp knife,
and put turpentine and mustard mixed together, to the wound;
keep putting this on until the wound runs matter ; then put
warm poultices to it.—(See pages 68 and 69.) At the same
time bleed from the arm, and repeat the bleeding according
to the state of the pulse. Put leeches all along the back-bone,
and when the leeches drop off, put the patient into a warm
bath and keep the leech-bites bleeding for some time, with
flannels wrung out in hot water. Then give this, if a grown
person, less according to the age ;—15 grains of calomel, and
four of five hours afterward, a wineglassful of castor-oil, with
a teaspoonful of spirits of turpentine in it. If the medicine is
slow in operating, give clysters, until the bowels are well
emptied ; then give a teaspoonful of laudanum at one dose.
If this does not produce sleep or ease in half an hour, give
15 drops of laudanum every hour, until the patient is easy.
Should the disease prove obstinate, give tobacco injections ;
        A teaspoonful of snuff,
        To a pint of boiling water.
In desperate cases, you may try blisters from the back of the
13

neck to the fundament, and give spirits of turpentine in doses
of a teaspoonful every half hour. While the patient is taking
other remedies, give him good old wine freely. Sometimes
antimonial wine, in large doses, every hour or half hour,
may do good.—See page 46.

ASTHMA.

Symptoms.—A feeling as if a tight cord was across the
chest, great anxiety and difficulty of breathing, with a short,
dry cough. These symptoms soon increase; the breathing
becomes very laborious, and has a wheezing sound; the patient gasps, and has a feeling of suffocation, and his countenance shows great uneasiness and distress; he is apt to rush
to the window or door for fresh air. After a while, these
distressing symptoms gradually wear off, and the patient
spits up a quantity of clear mucus, and is relieved. The distressing symptoms are apt to return, however, and are
always more severe during the night than during the day.

Treatment.—If the patient is young, strong, and hearty,
and you see the face look as if the blood is settling in it,
bleed moderately, and give this;

    3 grains of hippo,
    2 teaspoonfuls of vinegar,

to be given every quarter of an hour, until the patient is sick
at his stomach, or throws up. If the patient is affected with
a stoppage of water, or has swelled feet, or suffers constantly
with the disease, give this;

    A teaspoonful of pearlash;

pour on this vinegar, until it ceases to bubble up, and give a
half wineglass of the mixture every hour, until the urine
comes freely. If the fit is obstinate, give this;

    A teaspoonful of tincture of lobelia,

every ten minutes, until the patient is relieved. If the disease
is obstinate, and continues to annoy the patient from time to
time, great benefit may be derived from the Warm springs of
North Carolina. The patient should bathe frequently in the
spring, and avoid taking cold, eat simple food, and not eat too
much of that.

STOPPAGE OF THE MONTHLY COURSES,

WHILE they are flowing, or at the time when they are about to appear, frequently causes very serious, painful, and alarming affections, such as violent pains, like spasms in the bowels and stomach, and sometimes frequent retching to puke. Sometimes craziness, fits, and a loss, for a time, of motion or feeling. Sometimes, also, great difficulty in breathing, violent palpitations of the heart, or high fever and inflammation of the lungs, stomach, brain, or some other organ. Whenever, therefore, you observe any of these symptoms, after the courses have stopped, you may conclude that they have not been free enough, or just at the time when they ought to appear, you may conclude that they have been stopped, and proceed to this

Treatment.—If the patient is strong and hearty, and you see symptoms of a determination of blood to any organ, bleed, and purge out the bowels immediately with this ;

4 grains of calomel,
4 grains of rhubarb,
3 grains of aloes (powdered),

in one dose ; give a powder every two hours, until the bowels are emptied. Clysters are also very useful. The patient must be made to sit down in warm water, up to the hips, frequently. Bathe the feet frequently in warm water and mustard. If the pain in the lower part of the belly is very severe, give this, after the bowels have been well purged out ;

3 grains of powdered opium,
10 grains of camphor,

together, at one dose. Or, give this, as an injection ;

1 gill of thin starch,
1 teaspoonful of laudanum,
30 grains of camphor (powdered very fine).

But if the patient is feeble, with a weak and small pulse, you must try to strengthen the system with mild bitter tonics (see pages 64, 65, and 66), such as Columbo root, Peruvian bark, Gentian, and Port wine, and give mild nourishing food. The bowels must be opened, also, with mild purges, as castor-oil, or cream of tartar (see *Cathartics* in table), and kept gently open, and the patient take gentle exercise. Give this ;

40 grains of rhubarb,
15 grains of aloes,

rubbed up with a little white sugar, and made into eight

powders or pills, with gum Arabic.   Take one every night and morning.   Or this ;

    4 grains of green vitriol,
    5 grains of aloes,
    A little gum arabic,

rubbed together well, and made into ten pills or powders ; take one every morning and night.

PAINFUL AND DIFFICULT COURSES.

The treatment of this complaint must be of two kinds ; one to relieve the patient, while she is suffering from pain during her courses, the other to prevent a return of the suffering and cure the disease.

If the patient is suffering and is strong and healthy, bleed immediately, and let her sit down in warm water up to the hips, or even put her in a warm bath.   Next, inquire if the bowels are costive ; if so, give this ;

    8 grains of blue pill,
    4 grains of antimonial powder,

at one dose, and four or five hours afterward, a dose of castor-oil or Epsom salts.—(See table.)   As soon as the bowels are emptied, for if they are not by this, you must give injections (see page 70), give this ;

    5 grains of camphor,
    5 grains of Dover's powder,

rubbed up, and made into one powder ; give a powder every hour, until the pain is relieved.   The patient must drink freely of flaxseed or life-everlasting tea.   If the pain is obstinate, put large warm anodyne poultices over the womb, just above the hair of the privates.

To remove the disease when it is habitual, attend to these directions : If the patient is habitually costive, she must take, every now and then, a dose of blue pill, say five grains at night, and next morning a dose of castor-oil, Epsom salts, cream of tartar, or any mild purge.   She must eat light, digestible, vegetable food ; take gentle exercise by walking, but not ride on horseback.   Never let the bowels be costive.

Take every now and then, an emetic of hippo, when you go to bed.—(See page 46.) You may take this every now and then, also, on going to bed;

    2 grains of camphor,

    ₄ 2 grains of hippo,

rubbed together. You may try now and then, also (for it is generally an obstinate case), this;

    A teaspoonful of the ammoniated tinct. of guaiacum,

    1 teaspoonful of the wine of cochicum,

    A large glassful of sugar and water, boiled into syrup.

Take a tablespoonful three or four times a day. If these remedies fail, try this;

    1 grain of the extract of stramonium,

made into eight pills; give one pill three times a day. An apothecary or physician must make these pills. Various other remedies may be tried from time to time, as the senega acetate of potash, and many of the diuretics.—(See page 42 to page 45.) If all other means fail, salivate the patient by giving small doses of mercurial preparation.

THE WHITES.

This disease may be produced by various causes, as indolence and want of exercise, high living, excessive drinking, any irritation of the privates from child-birth, or the use of instruments in delivery, habitual costiveness, want of cleanliness, a general state of bad health, &c.

Treatment.—If the patient is strong and hearty, take a little blood every now and then, and purge the bowels out well with blue pill.—(See page 20.) Keep the bowels free, but do not purge too much. Make the patient sit down frequently in blood-warm water, and keep the privates clean, by washing frequently with castile soap, taking care not to rub them too much. Get from an apothecary, also, a *female* syringe, and use this;

    40 grains of alum,

    1 pint of the decoction of red-oak bark,

made in this way; take a tablespoonful of the red-oak bark,

13*

powdered; pour on it a pint of boiling water, and put in the alum. Syringe with this frequently. Or, you may try this;

A tumbler of rain-water,

20 drops of pyrolignous acid in it.

Syringe with this. Or this;

30 grains of white vitriol,

To 1 pint of water,

Give this, also, as a medicine after the bowels are opened;

8 grains of alum,

3 grains of hippo,

rubbed up into one powder; take one powder in the morning, and one in the evening, for several days.

If this fails, try 4 balsam copaiva capsules a day, one every three hours; and if they fail, try this; 20 drops of the tincture of cantharides, in water, three times a day, and increase the dose from day to day, until the water begins to burn, then stop, and go on again, after a while. Sometimes spirits of turpentine, ten drops, three times a day, may do good. If the patient is feeble and sickly, nourishing food, gentle exercise by walking, change of air, &c., and I have known benefit derived from the use of the nitro-muriatic bath.—(See page 68.) Lastly, try blisters to the back, just above the fundament.

CHLOROSIS, OR GREEN SICKNESS.

This disease is confined almost to young females, though it sometimes is seen in males.

Symptoms.—Face peculiarly pale, and of a somewhat swollen appearance; eyelids puffy, lips colorless. Frequently a dark, lead-colored streak under the lower eyelids, or the whole of the eyelids of greenish yellow hue. As the disease advances, the body begins to pine away, the feet, ankles, and legs, swell; the hands and fingers become white, puffy, and flabby, and sometimes the whole body becomes pale. Tongue pale, and covered with a transparent slime, looks swollen; and you will see marks of the teeth indented on it. Breath offensive; headache, ringing noise in the ears, giddiness, and the patient not inclined to exert herself, and often fretful and ill-tempered. Several other symptoms appear at times.

This disease is apt to be complicated with the whites, and is often produced by it, or excessive.flow of the courses ; or it may arise from indolent habits, unwholesome food and air, the courses not appearing at the proper time, neglected costiveness, and chronic irritation of the bowels. In this disease, when long continued, the patient is apt to have a craving for such things as chalk, ashes, clay, &c.

Treatment.—If the bowels are costive, and the belly swollen and tight, as they are apt to be, keep them open with this :

 4 grains of rhubarb,
 2 grains of aloes,

rubbed together, and given at one dose at night. Give one of these powders every third night, until the bowels are well emptied and loose. Give this, also, once or twice a week :

 5 grains of blue pill,
 1 grain of the extract of hyosciamus,

made into one pill. Nourishing and light food, as broths, game; change of air, gentle exercise, and sea-bathing in warm weather. When the disease has lasted some time, try this :—

 30 grains of green vitriol,
 A teaspoonful of white sugar,

rubbed up and made into six powders; give one powder every morning and evening; or this :—

 24 grains of the black sulphuret of iron,
 A teaspoonful of white sugar,

made into three powders; give one powder three times a day. The citrate of iron is a beautiful preparation, but I have never tried it. I have used the following pills with much benefit :—

 6 grains of calomel,
 6 grains of Kermes' mineral,
 18 grains of gum-guaiacum,

made into six pills; give one pill every morning.and night.

JAUNDICE.

SOMETIMES this disease comes on slowly, and with distinct symptoms, such as a general feeling of weariness, and an aversion to move about; peevishness and melancholy, costiveness, bad appetite, belching of acid stuff, slight wind-pains in the bowels, fullness and tightness at the pit of the stomach, oppression of the chest, restlessness at night, chills every now and then, with flushes of heat, sick stomach, and the urine is muddy, and deposites a thick stuff like pitch. After a few days, the skin begins to itch all over, the taste in the mouth is bitter, the urine of a deep-yellow color, the passages whitish or clay-colored. The whites of the eyes and skin about the lips, neck, and forehead, next become yellow, and afterward the whole body. Or the eyes and skin may become yellow without any particular symptoms. Again, it may come on in this way: a severe pain all at once, just below and to the right of the pit of the stomach. This soon increases, becomes very painful, and extends to the left shoulder, the loins, and all about the stomach; sickness at the stomach, and violent puking.

The color of the skin in jaundice is not always the same, but sometimes it is yellow, like gold, sometimes a greenish yellow, and sometimes dark or almost black. When it is greenish or dark, the liver is generally diseased, and it is called black jaundice; when yellow, yellow jaundice. This disease may disappear in a short time, or become chronic and last for some time, and waste the patient away, or kill him. The black jaundice is the most dangerous. Gall-stones are apt to be formed in the gall-bladder, and when they are coming away they give excruciating pain, but the patient is generally better afterward.

Treatment.—If there is great pain about the stomach, bleed immediately, if the patient can bear it. Then put him into a warm bath, and when you take him out, put leeches to the place where the pain is, and when they drop off, put warm poultices to the leech-bites.—(See page 69.) Then give this, if a grown person :—

    4 grains of powdered opium,
    15 grains of calomel,

rubbed together, and given at one dose. If this does not purge out the bowels quickly, give clysters until they are (see page 70). Put the patient several times into a warm bath. When the bowels are well emptied, feel the pulse; if you find it slow, full, and rather active, give an emetic of hippo, or two or three of them, until the patient throws up freely, when gall-stones are very apt to come away. But if the pulse is small, quick, and tight, like a cord, and the skin warm and dry, you may know that one of the guts, called the duodenum, is inflamed, and you must then put blisters to the pit of the stomach, and when the blister comes off, put warm poultices to the raw place (see page 69). Give this :—

        3 grains of Dover's powder,

every two hours; keep the bowels open with clysters, and the patient must take cool acid drinks, as lemonade, and gruel or boiled milk for nourishment. Emetics or purges here would be wrong. Lastly, when the disease is not very violent, but obstinate, and lasts for some time, keep the bowels open with a dose of blue pill or calomel every now and then, followed by some mild purge (see page 20), and pay particular attention to the patient's food and clothing.

FLATULENT OR WIND COLIC.

THIS may arise from two causes : indigestible food eaten in too great quantity, or a chronic irritation of the coats of the stomach and some of the bowels. When it arises from the first cause, the symptoms are these : a feeling of distention and uneasiness in the pit of the stomach, or a little below, on the left side. This feeling of distention of the stomach and bowels soon increases very much, with a dull, sickening pain. All these pains soon become very severe, and particularly about the navel. The patient generally tosses, rolls, or moves about quickly, with his body bent forward, and both hands pressed against his belly. If the colic is confined principally to the stomach, the patient will belch up a great quantity of wind; but if it is in one of the large guts, called the colon, the wind passes downward, but with much more difficulty, and frequently not until the patient has been relieved by medicine, &c. To distinguish colic from inflammation of the bowels, notice this : the patient is relieved by pressure on his belly (see *Inflammation of the Stomach*, page 104, and *Inflammation of the Bowels*, page 106), so that you may not mistake one disease for the other. You must not confound it with *bilious* colic, neither, for in bilious colic there is a puking of bile, and the eyes are yellowish, headache, and bitter taste in the mouth, which is not the case in flatulent colic. And you can easily distinguish it from paint-er's colic, for painter's colic comes on slowly, but this very quickly and violently. It is not generally a dangerous com-plaint, but requires immediate relief, as it may produce in-flammation of the bowels.

Treatment.—When it comes on just after the patient has eaten heartily, give a teaspoonful of hippo in warm water, with twenty drops of the essence of peppermint in it, for a grown person. If this does not puke, give another dose. About a quarter of an hour after the patient has puked, if his stomach is settled, give this :—

> A large wineglass of castor-oil,
> With 30 drops of the spirits of turpentine;

and, if this does not purge in two or three hours, give clys-ters, until the bowels are well emptied (see page 70). Some-times the pain is so severe that the patient can not take medi-cine, or lie still. In that case, give this :—

> A teaspoonful of laudanum,
> 5 grains of camphor,

rubbed up with a little white sugar, and put into a wineglass of warm water. Give this at one dose. After this, you must always purge the bowels out as soon as the stomach will bear it, with this :—

> 8 grains of calomel,
> 15 grains of jalap,

at one dose. If the patient is very strong and hearty, and the medicines are slow in operating, you must bleed. After all the pains and severe symptoms have been removed, the bowels well purged out, &c., if the part about the pit of the stomach is tender when you press it, and the tongue red at the edges, and with a fur in the middle, you must put leeches over the stomach or a blister, and afterward warm poultices, and if the inflammation is obstinate, follow the directions for acute inflammation of the stomach (see page 104). When colic is not severe, and arises from chronic irritation of the stomach and bowels, it will be only necessary to rub the belly well with a brush or dry flannels, and give this :—

> From 5 to 10 grains of camphor (well powdered),
> 30 drops of vitriolic ether,
> 30 drops of laudanum,

in a little warm water and sugar.

BILIOUS COLIC.

Premonitory Symptoms.—A bitter taste in the mouth, headache, loss of appetite, sick stomach, thirst, and sometimes puking of bile. After these, a sharp pain, sometimes very severe, is felt particularly about the navel; the pain generally moves about from one place to another, in the bowels. There is generally considerable sickness at the stomach, and puking of bile, from the commencement of the attack, and the bowels can be pressed upon without pain, but they generally become tender afterward. Patient generally relieved for a time by the puking; bowels generally very costive from the commencement of the attack. Sometimes one of the first symptoms is a yellowness of the skin and eyes, but more frequently this does not come on until about the second or third day of the disease.

Treatment.—If there is much sickness of the stomach, and the patient does not puke freely, give a dose of tartar-emetic, or two, if necessary (see page 46). If, however, he pukes very freely, let him drink freely of warm camomile or flaxseed tea. Next, cover the bowels with warm mustard-poultices (see p. 68), or put on a blister, if necessary, and when it makes the place red, take it off, and then put on the mustard-poultices (see page 68). When the stomach has been well emptied, and is settled, or as soon as you can get it down, give this : a half a grain of calomel, in a little sugar and water, every half hour; this will settle the stomach. As soon as the stomach is settled, give this :—

15 grains of calomel,

and about three hours afterward, a wineglass of castor-oil, if a grown person. If the medicine is thrown up, as is apt to be the case, you must give this : 5 grains of calomel every three hours, giving at the same time a purgative clyster (see page 70), until the bowels are well purged out; then give a full dose of opium (see page 29). If all these fail, you must give the calomel and opium pills, one every hour (see page 71), until the gums are sore. The bowels must be kept constantly open, during the whole attack, by castor-oil, clysters, or a dose of calomel every now and then. Two or three passages a day will be sufficient.

If, at the commencement of the disease, the patient is

strong and healthy, and you see symptoms of a fullness of
blood in the system, called plethora, you must bleed, particularly if the pulse is strong and tight, like a cord, or the belly
is tender when you press on it.   This may be repeated from
time to time, if the pulse and other symptoms indicate it.
The warm bath is very useful every now and then.   When
the patient is recovering, particular care is necessary to prevent a return of the disease, from eating anything unwholesome, or taking cold.   Put a flannel bandage around the
belly, and let the patient wear it for some time, and give
for nourishment rice-gruel, sage-tea, chicken-water, &c.

PAINTER'S COLIC.

This is sometimes called the dry gripes.   It is always
caused by the poisonous influence of lead in some way.

Symptoms.—It generally comes on slowly, with costiveness, belching disagreeable air, sick stomach, weariness,
drowsiness, and a disinclination to exertion of mind or body,
a feeling of weight and tightness, with occasional wandering
pains in the belly.   These symptoms generally increase, and
the pain about the pit of the stomach and the navel gradually increases; the belly becomes hard, and tender on pressure, the bowels very costive, and the stomach generally very
irritable.   A great many other symptoms may appear, particularly in severe cases, as cold sweats of the hands and
feet, pale face, convulsions.

Treatment.—If the pulse is strong and full, bleed immediately until the patient is sick, and then give this :—

   5 grains of calomel,
   2 grains of powdered opium,

made into one powder, and given every two hours until the
pain is relieved.   When the pain is relieved, give this :—

   3 grains of calomel,
   ½ grain of powdered opium,

made into one powder, and give every three hours, until the
gums are sore.   As soon as the gums are sore, give this :—

   A wineglass of castor-oil,
   2 teaspoonfuls of spirits of turpentine,

given at one dose : if this does not purge in three hours, give half this dose every hour, until the bowels are well purged out. After the bowels have been well purged out, if the pains return, you must give the calomel and opium powders again, as directed, every three or four hours, until the patient is salivated. Should the powders have no effect, give purgative clysters, until the bowels are well emptied.—(See page 70.) Should all these remedies fail to relieve the pain in the belly, give this :—

     20 grains of alum (powdered),
      1 grain of opium (powdered),

made into one powder, and given every three or four hours, until relieved. After this, you must again give a dose of castor-oil, and one of calomel and opium, as recommended, every now and then, and keep the bowels open with clysters. When the patient is getting better, he must take chicken water, and meat broths, and be careful not to drink cold water or spirits. Diluent drinks must be given.—(See page 39.)

CHOLERA-MORBUS.

THIS is produced by the same cause as flatulent colic, and in fact, is the same, only that in the latter, the violent pains are prevented, and the patient relieved by the puking and purging which takes place.

Symptoms.—Sickness at the stomach, every now and then, and belching acid, disagreeable stuff. Cutting pains in the bowels, particularly screwing pains about the navel. These symptoms generally come on at night, after the patient has been a little while in bed, or asleep. The bowels rumble frequently, and the patient soon begins to puke and purge rapidly, a sour, disagreeable stuff, in which you can detect the unwholesome food, which was the cause.

Treatment.—Give an emetic of hippo immediately (see page 46), and as soon as the patient's stomach is settled, give a dose of castor-oil and laudanum.—(See page 71.) Should the stomach be too weak for the castor-oil, give two of the

14

calomel and opium pills (see page 71), and repeat them until the patient is relieved. Put cataplasms or warm mustard poultices to the belly.—(See page 68.) Should the disease prove obstinate, follow the directions for flatulent colic.—(See page 154.)

CHOLERA OF INFANTS.

THIS disease generally occurs in children, between three months and two years of age.

Symptoms.—It generally comes on gradually; you will observe a looseness of the bowels for several days, when the child begins to puke. The passages are generally frothy, or watery, or whitish, or thin and colorless. The child is apt to die in a few days, but if not, it generally wastes away; hands and feet become cold, head and belly hot; the face pale and shrunk, or pinched, the eyes dull and sunken, skin dry, pulse small, irritated, and quick. If the child now does not get better, it becomes sleepy, lies with its eyes half open when asleep, and rolls its head about when awake, and, at last, becomes insensible, as if in apoplexy, or goes off in convulsions.

Treatment.—If the child is teething, and the gums swollen, cut them. Next, put ten or twelve leeches behind the ears, or to the temples; I prefer behind the ears; make the bites bleed freely, with flannels wrung out in hot water, and then put a blister the size of a dollar, or larger, according to the size of the child, behind the ears, over the leech-bites. Next give this:—

> 2 grains of calomel,
> 6 grains of hippo,

well rubbed together, and made into twelve powders. Give one powder in a little sugar and water every hour; or, if the child is not very ill, every two hours, and keep on giving them until the passages look good, and you see bile in them. Then you can stop and keep the bowels open with moderate doses of castor-oil.—(See page 33.)   Regulate the dose according to the age of the child—for a child three months old, a teaspoonful of the best oil (give none but the best).   At the same time that you commence giving the powder, cover the child's whole belly with warm mustard poultices (see page 58), and when the skin is made quite red, put on simple warm poultices instead, frequently.   Every now and then, when you go to change a poultice, you must put the child into a warm bath, and while it is in the water, put cold wet cloths to the head. If, however, the child is very sick, lose no time, but put a large blister over the pit of the stomach, and let it cover a little lower down.   When the blister has been on about four hours, if the place is quite red (that is, if the blister has drawn, it must not draw until it makes bladders), take it off, and cover the whole of the bowels from the pit of the stomach to near the privates with a warm mustard poultice (see page 68), the quantity of mustard in the poultice, according to the age of the child.   As soon as the bladders have risen well, take off the poultice and dress the place with a rag spread with fresh mercurial ointment, and repeat the dressings to keep the place running.   If the powders which I have directed, do not open the bowels enough, or seem to be too slow, give one grain of calomel every hour (for a young child), until they are ; and then go on with the powders.   If after the violence of the disease has been subdued, the child remains emaciated, with a dry, shrunk skin, &c., give this (that is, if you see no symptoms of a determination of blood to the head, as sleepiness, &c.) :—

> 1 grain of calomel,
> 3 grains of Dover's powder,
> 1 grain of rhubarb,

made into six powders; give one powder every two hours, or you may put a quarter of a grain of sulphate of morphine, in place of the Dover's powder.   Sometimes when the child is slowly getting better, it is distressed with wind pains in the bowels.   To relieve these, give two drops of the spirits of turpentine, in a little boiled milk, every one or two hours. If this does not answer, give this—a teaspoonful of common soot, pour on it a wineglassful of water, strain it, and sweeten with white sugar; give a teaspoonful every half hour or so. During the whole course of the disease, the child must have, for nourishment, nothing but a little boiled milk, or thin arrow-root, or rice gruel; when it is very weak, you may give beef-tea, or chicken water. If the child is nursing, the milk is the best nourishment

Lastly ; if the disease is obstinate, try change of air, to some warm, dry place, put on flannel, and let the child have exercise, and fresh air, in mild weather. Keep woollen stockings to the feet.

SLIPPING OF ONE GUT INTO ANOTHER, CALLED ILIUS, OR ILIAC PASSION.

THIS accident, and consequent disease, may be produced by various causes; as powerful emetics, or purges, indigestible food, green fruit, and any hard substances swallowed accidentally, which clog the passages of the guts, violent cholera-morbus, and puking, or colic. Again, it may arise from wounds in the belly, hernia (or rupture), &c. It is one of the most difficult diseases to discover by symptoms at its first attack ; for the symptoms are, at times, very like those of flatulent colic (see page 153), or cholera-morbus (see page 157), or spasms of the belly. By careful attention, however, to these symptoms which follow, you may detect it ; and if you happen to mistake it for colic, the treatment will be tolerably correct.

Symptoms.—Sometimes, but rarely, it comes on slowly and insidiously, taking months, or a longer time, before it is developed; but it usually comes on suddenly, like flatulent colic, without any warning. Violent spasms and pains in the belly, belching up winds, belly puffed out; the patient tosses about, and tries frequently to have a passage, but can not, and you may see all the symptoms which occur as flatulent colic. After these symptoms, the bowels becomes obstinately costive, and if you give injections, the passages which come away are mixed with, or composed entirely of clotted blood. Sometimes hiccough, and puking what may be in the stomach, and even dung. If you feel different parts of the belly, you are apt to find a hard, irregular swelling, shaped like a gut, folded back and forward, which is the place where a part of

COSTIVENESS. 161

one gut has slipped into another, like a glove-finger drawn off hastily, or a small gut into a large one.

Treatment.—As soon as the patient is attacked, examine him and see if he has hernia (or rupture, as it is commonly called), if so, push it up. If the pulse is full and hard, and the patient strong and hearty, bleed freely. Next, give this, if a grown person:—

          10 grains of calomel,
           1 grain powdered opium,

made into one dose, and given in a little syrup. If this does not relieve the pain, give this:—

          5 grains of camphor,
          2 grains of opium,

rubbed up with a little white sugar, and given in a little warm water or syrup. You must lose no time, but keep giving injections (purgative clysters, see page 70), until you get one or two good passages, when you may conclude that the gut has slipped out again, or the contraction and spasm removed. If, however, you do not get passages quickly, keep giving ten grains of calomel every now and then, followed in a quarter of an hour by a teaspoonful of castor-oil, and give the castor-oil in these doses, every quarter of an hour. Put the patient also, into a warm bath, every now and then. Lastly, if you can not succeed in getting passages, give emetics of hippo, in large doses (see page 46), cover the bowels with warm mustard poultices (page 68), or blisters dressed with the mustard poultices, and keep throwing warm water up the fundament with a forcing injection apparatus; pump up a whole basinful, if you can, or more. Do not let your patient die for want of exertion to get purges through him, or clysters, or from neglecting any means to give relief, and loosen the gut, as emetics, warm bath, quicksilver, an ounce or more at a dose. Tobacco injections may be tried.

* * *

COSTIVENESS.

This is too often neglected, and may give rise to ill-health, or serious and dangerous diseases, or it may lead to such disagreeable and disgusting results, as to make life a burthen, as ill-temper, hypochondria, dyspepsia, piles, bad breath, &c.

14*

The means by which it may be prevented or removed when it is habitual, are the following :—Never neglect trying every day; take exercise on foot or horseback. If you are a female and in a family way, take a dose of castor-oil every now and then ; it will give you an easy time in labor. Take your meals regularly, and do not eat as much as your appetite will let you. Eat such things as these—vegetables well boiled, hard biscuits, brown bread ; eat a very little meat, and let that be game, or the meat of old animals, as beef-steak, mutton, poultry, and these rather rare. Never remain too long without eating, and take a little walk after each meal. Ripe fruit is wholesome, also good olive oil, eaten frequently with your meals. But avoid such articles as the following: fresh bread, highly-seasoned dishes, as hashes and French condiments, pies and pastry, cinnamon and nutmegs, cabbages, turnips, salad, &c. Should the habit be obstinate, you must use the soap as directed in page 70, or a mild clyster every morning when you wake.—(See page 70.) If these fail, take this :—

    40 grains of blue pill, mass,
     6 grains of powdered aloes,

well rubbed up, and made into six pills, one or two every night if necessary. Or if these do not open the bowels sufficiently, take every morning early, besides, a moderate wine-glassful of the compound tincture of rhubarb. Should all these means fail, you must give from five to eight grains of blue pill, with the same quantity of the compound extract of colocynth, every night and morning, and continue these until the patient's gums are sore, using an injection every morning, also.

———

HÆMORRHOIDS, COMMONLY CALLED PILES.

THESE are of two kinds, which will be described as follows:
Symptoms.—A feeling of weight and tightness about the hips, and near the opening of the fundament. This feeling usually goes off in three or four days ; after a while, however, it returns, and you will notice very red blood on the surface of your passages, but not mixed up with them. This pain and these symptoms may appear and disappear from time to

time when you will notice tumors, or risings, of various sizes, sometimes large and sometimes small, and painful or otherwise, inside, or just about the orifice of the fundament. This is one kind. The swellings are of a dark color, and bluish, soft when you touch them; are lessened in size when you press them, but quickly return to their former size when you remove your fingers. These tumors are generally found in clusters, and extend some way up the fundament. These are called the blind piles.

Another kind are of a pale-red or brownish color, look like small fleshy warts, or hang down from the orifice of the fundament; they feel hard and spongy. These tumors appear generally to be filled with blood, and are apt to become dark after a while. Several other symptoms, besides those which I have described, are apt to appear just before the piles make their appearance. Frequently also there is a discharge from these piles, which is very disagreeable.

Treatment of the Blind Piles.—Wash them every now and then with cold water, particularly after having a passage. If they are up the fundament, use with care an injection of cold water, with a little Castile soap dissolved in it; and put a soft piece of lint over the orifice of the fundament, which must be kept from slipping by a cross bandage fastened to a band above the hips. If the piles become inflamed and give much pain, you must apply soft poultices, sprinkled over with lead-water (about four grains of sugar of lead dissolved in a wineglass of water). Or apply anodyne poultices (see page 68), and if the piles are outside, scarify them with a lancet, and let them bleed well. The bowels must be kept loose, but not purging, with mild medicines.— (See page 30, *Aperients.)* If there is a discharge of white matter from the fundament, as sometimes happens, use carefully injections of this :—

    1 grain of blue vitriol,
    In a wineglass of cold water.
Or this :—
    2 grains of sugar of lead,
    In a wineglass of cold water.
If the piles are outside, and give much trouble after this, they must be cut off with a knife.

DIARRHŒA, OR LOOSENESS OF THE BOWELS, CALLED BY SOME, BOWEL-COMPLAINT.

Symptoms.—Large, loose passages frequently, with griping, but no straining, as in dysentery, and no fever. When, however, the disease lasts a long time, there is apt to be a slight fever toward evening, or a short time after eating; the skin becomes dry and harsh, the pulse small, quick, and irritated; the body wastes away, and the feet and legs generally swell, or water is formed on the bowels. The patient is apt also to feel severe pains like colic, wind in the bowels, and to have discharges from the bowels just after eating, and frequently you see pieces of food in the passages but half digested. The passages are sometimes slimy, or abundant and watery; sometimes dark, reddish, or whitish.

This disease may be produced by various causes, as indigestible food and drink, unwholesome bile and secretions in the bowels, or acid in the stomach or bowels, acid fruit, &c. Some persons, however, are particularly liable to it, from a natural weakness of the bowels. It is also very frequently produced by cold and exposure in damp, rainy weather. And it arises sometimes, again, from the same causes which produce dysentery, as cool, damp nights in the fall after a hot day. When it arises from this last, you will generally observe the following symptoms before the disease comes on: a weight and uneasiness about the chest, a feeling of fullness and tightness in the belly, bitter taste in the mouth, and bad appetite, headache, and disturbed sleep, creeping chills every now and then, slight weariness, and aching pain in the back.

Treatment.—The treatment of this disease must depend upon the cause which produced it, and must be varied from time to time, according to the symptoms. As a general rule, follow these directions: when the disease is of recent occurrence, that is to say, before it has run on so long as to become somewhat habitual, open the bowels with this:—

A tablespoonful of castor-oil,
5 drops of laudanum,

four times a day. At night give this:—

2 grains of calomel,
2 grains of hippo. And next morning—
5 grains of rhubarb,
3 grains of Dover's powder.

If the looseness of the bowels is not now checked, give this: a calomel and opium pill every three hours (see page 71) until bedtime; then stop, and if the patient is not relieved, give him warm flaxseed or starch clysters (see page 70), and put warm anodyne poultices over the whole of his bowels (see page 68). This treatment is especially proper when the disease is produced by cold and exposure. If the disease has lasted for some time, and the discharges from the bowels are great, you must give one or two moderate doses of castor-oil, until you find that the bowels are emptied. Then give this:—

  16 grains of blue pill,
  1 grain of the sulphate of morphine,

well rubbed together, and made into four pills: give one pill every three hours, and if the bowels are not checked, go on until the gums are a little sore; then give a moderate dose of castor-oil. If the disease has just commenced, and you see symptoms of bile, and acrid substances in the bowels, which is apt to be the case when the disease comes on from cool nights in the fall, and which you can discover by observing the symptoms described on page 164, give a moderate dose of the best castor-oil, and when it has operated, give these pills:—

  12 grains of hippo,
  3 grains of powdered opium,
  4 grains of calomel,

and just enough of the conserve of roses to make pills; rub them up well together, and divide into twelve pills: give one pill every two hours until bedtime; then stop, and if the bowels are not checked, go on again with the pills. Or you may give this after the oil has operated:—

  2 grains of calomel,
  A little white sugar,

rubbed up and made into eight powders; give one powder every two hours, or every hour if necessary. If the patient is a young child, give this:—

  1 grain of calomel,
  6 grains of crabs'-eyes,
  A little white sugar,

rubbed well together and made into six powders; give one powder every two hours. If the disease becomes obstinate

and chronic, and the patient wastes away, as is very apt to
be the case, give this :—

    24 grains of Dover's powder,
     3 grains of sugar of lead,
    A little white sugar,

well rubbed together, and made into four or five powders;
give one powder every three or four hours. If this fails to
check the bowels, see page 112, and follow the directions
for the treatment of chronic inflammation of the mucous membrane of the bowels.

INDIGESTION, OR DYSPEPSIA.

This complaint may arise from various sources, as eating
indigestible food, eating too much at a meal, eating too fast,
eating meals irregularly, chewing tobacco, drinking, not
chewing the food sufficiently, depressing and harassing emotions, a sedentary life, &c.

Symptoms.—It would be impossible to enumerate all the
symptoms which attend or precede this disease. The most
important, however, are the following: variable, weak, or
total loss of appetite, at the commencement of the disease;
wind in the bowels, and colic pains, belching acid stuff;
spirits depressed and gloomy; a constant uneasy feeling at
the pit of the stomach, and a craving of food at times, but
suffering and uneasiness after eating; weariness, or a languid
and relaxed state of the whole system, particularly a short
time after eating; bowels bound, or not sufficiently free, and
tongue covered generally with a white fur; various other
symptoms, also, as a feeling of choking and sinking at the
stomach, &c. These symptoms differ also, or others may
appear in different subjects, according as the disease is produced by one or the other of the causes which I have stated
as giving rise to it. This disease, also, is of two forms: one
in which the digestive organs appear to be merely sluggish,
as when the disease arises from inactive life, irregular meals,
overloading the stomach, &c. When this is the case, you
will see the following

Symptoms.—Tongue covered with a white fur, bad appetite, costiveness, belching acid and disagreeable stuff, pulse

not much altered, and no tenderness about the pit of the stomach, wind and colic in the bowels every now and then.

Treatment of the first Form of the Disease.—Attend to the directions in regard to your meals, laid down in page 162, for costiveness, with this exception, eat no vegetables. By strict attention to these directions, you may have your health quickly restored. If, however, your digestion remains obstinately weak, and you do not experience relief, particularly if your bowels are costive, take this :—

8 grains of rhubarb,
2 grains of aloes,

rubbed up with a little of the conserve of roses, and made into four pills; give one pill every night and morning, and take during the day some mild tonic, as wormwood, camomile-flowers, columbo-root, gentian, or some of the preparations of iron.—(See from page 64 to 67.)

The second form of dyspepsia is that in which there is inflammation and irritability of the digestive organs, and you will generally observe the following

Symptoms.—A red, somewhat marked or creased tongue, with little pimples or granules all over it, and sometimes glossy or shining; tenderness at the pit of the stomach and near by, when you press on it; a small, somewhat hard and quick pulse, and slight fevers or irritability of the system toward evening; body and face thin, bowels irregular, with loose, slimy, watery, or bilious passages every now and then; sometimes severe pain just below the pit of the stomach, a little after eating, &c.

Treatment.—With regard to the treatment of this form of dyspepsia, you must pay especial and particular attention to the directions given for chronic inflammation of the mucous membrane of the bowels (page 112), as it is pretty much the same disease. If the eyes and skin are yellowish, the urine and the passages have bile in them, as is frequently the case, give this :—

30 grains of blue pill,
10 grains of aloes,

rubbed well together, and made into ten pills; give one pill every other night until the symptoms of bile are removed. Use this every now and then also: ½ pint of flaxseed-tea, made a little slimy; put in four grains of saltpetre, and give a wineglass, when cold, every hour or two during the day.

Use flaxseed and starch clysters also every now and then.—
(See page 70.) In either form of the disease, if you see the
symptoms of bile which I have described, you may give
small doses of blue pill, with a little opium or morphine.
Use this :—

              12 grains of blue pill,
               2 grains of powdered opium,
rubbed together, and made into four pills ; give one pill every night.   Or these :—

               2 grains of blue pill,
               ¼ grain of sulphate of morphine,
made into one pill and taken every night.   Be careful not
to salivate, or even to make the gums sore.   Stop with the
pills every now and then.   If all these fail, and the patient
gets no better, carry him to Aiken, or the warm springs of
North Carolina, not forgetting the directions about food, clothing, &c.

HOOPING COUGH.

Symptoms.—This disease generally commences with the
usual symptoms of cold, such as uneasiness and difficulty of
breathing, slight hoarseness, sneezing, and headache ; bowels costive, appetite weak, patient a little feverish toward
evening, and starts in its sleep.   Then a dry, ringing cough
begins, which lasts for two or three weeks generally ; the fits
of coughing are at this time generally short, and there is no
hooping.   After a while, however, the fits of coughing become more frequent, and last a longer time ; the child expe-
riences great difficulty during the fits, in catching its breath,
from the closure of the neck of the windpipe, and you will
hear a peculiar, loud, hooping noise, every time it draws its
breath in coughing, which can not be mistaken.   Notice this
also : just before a fit of coughing comes on, the patient feels
a tickling in the throat and chest, and a tightness in the breast,
as if a cord was tied around the chest ; which symptoms will
enable you to distinguish it from any other cough.   Very
frequently, just after a fit of coughing, the child spits up a
quantity of clear, slimy stuff, or mucus, and sometimes pukes.
The fits of coughing last longer in some cases than in others.

Sometimes they are very short, and sometimes long and very severe, and the child will turn purple in the face, or seem to suffocate ; sometimes convulsions come on, or blood will gush from the mouth and nose. The disease also may last a fortnight, or four and six weeks, before it begins to abate. This is a very contagious or catching disease, but not often dangerous, unless very severe, or the child catches a cold. It may be taken, but not often, by grown persons, and you never have it twice.

Treatment.—If the pulse is full and strong, bleed, and if there is much pain and oppression at the chest, put leeches over the chest and to the pit of the stomach. When the fits of coughing are very severe and the patient is much distressed, put your finger down the throat, so as to make it puke ; if this does not succeed, you must give an emetic of white vitriol (see page 47), or of hippo (see page 46) ; and to relieve the cough, give this : one pint of flaxseed-tea, made a little slimy, with one grain of tartar emetic in it. Give a wineglass of this every hour, when cold. Or this :—

A teaspoonful of the syrup of squills,
1   do.   antimonial wine,
1   do.   paregoric,
2   do.   spirits of nitre ;

take two wineglasses of boiling water, dissolve a little liquorice in the water, and mix them all together. Give a teaspoonful of this every hour or two. You may try this also :

1 teaspoonful of vinegar of squills,
1 tablespoonful of the emulsion of asafœtida,

made by pouring a wineglass of boiling water on 15 grains of asafœtida ; mix them together, and give a teaspoonful in the same manner. Various other remedies may be used, when the cough is very violent, as syrup of poppies, hippo in small doses, lobelia inflata, belladonna, &c. When the disease is mild, it will, in general, be only necessary to pay particular attention to the patient's food and clothing, and keep it from exposure, or catching cold. Change of air is generally beneficial in this disease ; and the air of Aiken being dry and light, peculiarly suitable.

15

WORMS.

The worms which inhabit the human system are of several kinds, but that which we most frequently meet with is the long round worm, which varies from two to ten or twelve inches in length, and are of a dingy-white or reddish-brown color, and larger in the middle of the body than at the two ends.

Symptoms.—It is a difficult matter to determine the presence of worms in the system by symptoms; but the symptoms which generally appear are the following: pains in the belly, generally about the navel; bowels bound, or frequent and slimy passages ; face pale or lead-colored, with the cheeks flushed every now and then ; eyes heavy and dull, with a bluish mark under the lower eyelids ; upper lip swelled, and the child picks at its nose frequently ; tongue covered with a fur or slime ; belly swelled and hard, dwindling away of the body, fretful temper, and sometimes a voracious appetite. Other symptoms may also appear. One of the most certain symptoms is the constant picking at the nose. It must be borne in mind, however, that a child may have worms without any of these symptoms, and the first indication is seeing them in the passages. Worms also occasion a great many alarming complaints, as convulsions or fits, dropsy, delirium or craziness, &c. All the complaints, however, are generally cured as soon as the worms come away.

Treatment.—Open the bowels well with this : a tablespoonful of castor-oil, with five drops of spirits of turpentine, every three or four hours, until the child has two or three passages (this is for a child five or six years old). Continue this treatment for two or three days ; then give this :—

A wineglassful of the pinkroot (broken up),
put into a pint of boiling water and boil down to a half-pint. Sweeten this and give a wineglassful every hour, for a child from five to eight or ten years. About an hour after the last dose, give this :—

2 tablespoonfuls of castor-oil,
1 teaspoonful of spirits of turpentine   Or this :—
5 grains of calomel,
3 grains of jalap,
3 grains of rhubarb,

rubbed up, and made into one or two doses, according to the age of the patient. If this does not bring away worms, try this :—

    10 grains of calomel,
    15 grains of powdered pink-root (spigelia),
    15 grains of rhubarb,

well rubbed together, and made into five powders; give one powder in the morning, one at midday, and one at evening, for a child ten years old ; two of the powders a day for one younger. This treatment must be persevered in for several days; and, to prevent the calomel from salivating, give the calomel, pink-root, and rhubarb powders, every other day, instead of every day, and on the odd or intervening days give the castor-oil and turpentine, as directed. Should this fail, which does not often happen, see pages 25 and 26, and try some of the medicines mentioned there. The child, while it is taking these medicines, must take nothing but very light or liquid food, as corn or rice gruel, or meat-soups, but no vegetables. Little negroes are much improved, and the expulsion of worms assisted, by giving them a little good fat bacon, fried, to eat.

ASCARIDES.

THESE are very small white worms, which are found about the fundament, and cause a most distressing tickling and itching about the part, which are the symptoms by which you may discover them

Treatment.—Give two grains of calomel at night, for a child ten years old, and the next morning give a clyster of this :—

    1 teaspoonful of spirits of turpentine,
    To a wineglass of warm milk.

Or this :—

    1 teaspoonful of powdered aloes ;

pour on this a wineglassful of boiling water, strain, and add when cool a wineglass of warm milk: inject with it. The injections must be repeated three times a day, and every other night give a dose of aloes, in powder, with sugar.—(See page

31.) Sometimes these little worms get into the privates of females. Then use this :—

> 1 teaspoonful of vinegar,
> A wineglass of cold water;

Syringe out the privates well with this, with a female syringe, which you can get at any apothecary's. If the patient is a grown person, use larger doses; or it may be necessary to purge out the bowels more frequently and more freely.

TAPE-WORM.

This is a long white worm; sometimes it is twenty, thirty, or forty feet in length, and is found in the stomach and upper bowels. It is composed of a great many joints, about the size of a gourd-seed, which the joints resemble somewhat. This worm is apt to come away in pieces.

Treatment.—A great many remedies have been recommended for the expulsion of this worm, and as they are not very frequently met with, my experience in the treatment for them is rather limited. I have, however, treated several cases in the following manner. As soon as a portion of the worm is seen in the passages, give this, if a grown person :—

> 10 grains of calomel,
> 10 grains of jalap,

rubbed up, and made into one or two doses; give one dose two hours after the other. As soon as the medicine begins to work, give a purgative clyster.—(See page 70.) When the bowels have been well emptied, let the patient have a good bowl of gruel, or beef-tea, or chicken-water, made very salt; and he must drink very freely of green tea for five or six hours. On the following day keep the bowels well open, by giving a teaspoonful of castor-oil with a teaspoonful of turpentine every three hours, and giving this injection every now and then :—

> A wineglass of warm milk,
> A teaspoonful of turpentine,
> A half-wineglass of sweet-oil,

well mixed. If this does not succeed in bringing away more

of the worm, repeat the medicines for three or four days. If this does not succeed, try some of the medicines mentioned in pages 25 and 26 *(Anthelmintics).*

There is another kind of tape-worm, which has no joints: the treatment for this is the same.

DROPSY OF THE CELLULAR TISSUE UNDER THE SKIN—CALLED ANASARCA.

Symptoms.—Drowsiness and sluggishness of the mind, pale or sallow skin; and when you press hard on the skin with your fingers, a pit or hole is left. The disease generally commences in the feet and legs, and then spreads over all or most of the body. It may proceed from cold and a check of perspiration, irritation of the bowels, weakness after illness, eruptive diseases struck in, long-continued diarrhœa, discharges of blood from different parts, &c. It is also frequently complicated with dropsy of the bowels, and is then a more serious disease, and frequently is seen in persons who have suffered much from country fevers, or live in unhealthy places.

Treatment.—If the disease is produced by continued and repeated country fevers, open the bowels with this:—

> 8 grains of calomel,
> 10 grains of jalap,

given at one dose, for a grown person. If the patient is strong, as soon as the bowels are well opened, give this: acetate of potash, as directed in the table (page 43), and give at the same time, every morning, or every other morning, a dose of cream of tartar (see page 32). The patient may drink freely also of such drinks as the following: flaxseed-tea, a pint, with four grains of antimonial powder, or a tablespoonful of antimonial wine, or twenty or thirty grains of saltpetre in it. If, after following this plan for five or six days, you see no improvement, try some of the medicines mentioned under the head of Diaphoretics, in the table, and also under the head of Diuretics. It is a good plan to return to the remedies which I have recommended first, every now and then. The same treatment is proper when the disease arises from cold, checked perspiration, &c. But if it is the

15*

consequence of long illness, or produced by any weakening complaint, as diarrhœa or flow of blood, or the patient is weak, you must not give large doses, but give the patient good wine, camphor, seneka, Dover's powder, &c. (see pages 14, 37, and 36). When you find that the cream of tartar gripes and produces small watery passages, with pain, stop it for a day or so, and give this:—

A teaspoonful of the bark of slippery elm;
pour on a pint of boiling water: give a wineglassful every hour.

DROPSY IN THE CHEST.

This disease generally comes on slowly, and water may have been in the chest some time before you notice the following

Symptoms.—A feeling of weight and tightness at the pit of the stomach or just above it; slight difficulty of breathing when the patient is standing up and standing still; and when he lies down, walks up stairs, or walks fast, a great suffocation and difficulty of breathing. He is apt to start in his sleep also, and become much alarmed; short, dry cough, particularly while lying down or walking fast, swelled feet, anxious, alarmed, and pale countenance; great thirst, irregular pulse, urine high-colored, with a sediment, and small in quantity. The patient generally prefers sitting up, or leaning his chin over a bench or chair, to lying down. Sometimes the water is only in one side of the chest, and may be produced by neglected pleurisy, &c., or, when in the whole chest, by high living and drinking, and a full state of the system.

Treatment.—If the pulse is full and hard, and the patient strong, bleed from the arm. Next, put a large blister over the chest, or between the shoulders, and purge out the bowels well with two or three doses of cream of tartar (see page 32). After the bowels have been well emptied, say five or six hours after the last passage, give this:—

20 grains of powdered squills,
60 grains (1 drachm) of saltpetre,
3 grains of calomel,

well rubbed together, and made into five powders; give one powder every three or four hours. If this makes the patient sick at the stomach or irritates the bowels, divide the powders in half and give them as before ; or, you may give this :—

10 grains of saltpetre,
5 grains of calomel,
2 grains of powdered opium,
5 grains of powdered squills,

rubbed together, and made into two powders ; give one powder in the morning, and the other in the evening. If the patient is weak and relaxed, as a female, after flooding, the courses long continued, &c., give this :—

3 grains of camphor,
2 grains of opium,
1 grain of powdered squills,
3 grains of calomel,

rubbed together, and made into six powders ; give one powder every hour. Continue this treatment for five or six days, and if the patient is not better, apply to a physician.

DROPSY IN THE BELLY, CALLED ASCITES.

This disease may be mistaken, in females, for pregnancy, but you may easily distinguish it from pregnancy by attending carefully to the following

Symptoms.—In dropsy in the belly, when the patient lies on her back, the belly falls, as it were, to one side, and you can notice a distinct tumor or swelling, on striking which with the ends of the fingers of one hand, while those of the other hand are place opposite, you will notice what is called a fluctuation, which is a feeling as if water was in a bladder or skin. When the patient lies on her back, also, the belly seems to flatten on the top, and press out at the sides. In this disease, the breathing of the patient is much oppressed, when lying down. There is a dry skin, thirst, the urine is small in quantity, and when the patient breathes, the hips and the belly seem to rise higher than the chest (notice this), which symptoms do not appear in pregnancy. When the disease is

far advanced, the feet are apt to become dropsical, and sometimes the greater portion of the body. This disease is generally brought on by the following causes : chronic inflammation of the peritoneum (the membrane which surrounds the
bowels of the abdomen)—(see page 119), disease of the liver
or spleen, long-continued indigestion, inflammation of the
liver, fever and ague of long standing, drinking to excess, &c.

Treatment.—Purge out the bowels, as directed for dropsy
of the chest (page 174). Put several leeches over the belly,
and when they drop off, cover the belly with a large blister,
and dress the place when the blister is taken off, with cloths
spread with mercurial ointment. Let the patient take the
acetate of potash, as directed for dropsy under the skin (page
173), and follow the directions given there for the drinks which
are to be taken. Remember also, what I said about the cream
of tartar, and purgatives, when they act too violently (see
page 174), attend to the directions. Lastly, if you find that
your patient is not getting better, give him small doses of
calomel and opium, or blue pill and morphine, until his gums
are a little sore, but do not salivate. When all medicines and
remedies fail, either in dropsy under the skin, or of the belly,
have the patient tapped. The food, during the whole course
of the disease, must be very light, as chicken water, rice
gruel, with boiled milk, &c., and when the patient is getting
better, he must wear a broad flannel bandage, a little tight,
around his whole belly.

DIABETES, OR EXCESSIVE FLOW OF URINE.

As this disease is of two forms, I will describe first, that
which is called *Sweet Diabetes,* and may be known by the
following

Symptoms.—The urine is generally in great quantity, of
a pale straw color, or sometimes of a greenish shade, sweet-
ish taste, and has a faint smell, like milk, or meat broths.
Tongue white and foul, or sometimes red and clean; bowels
generally costive ; pain and weakness in the loins ; pain
and some inflammation about the foreskin and head of the

privates in a man; great thirst, dry skin, mouth hot and dry, great appetite, and a feeling of weight and uneasiness about the stomach after eating. The patient is thin, weak, and dislikes exercise or exertion; headache, giddiness in the head, and confused and indistinct eyesight; pulse generally not much altered, except when the disease is far advanced, when it is sometimes very frequent and quick, and many other alarming symptoms appear, as drowsiness, great emaciation, &c.

This disease may last four or five weeks before the patient dies, or several months, or even years; and the patient may get better, and the disease return again and again. Some persons are much more liable to it than others. This disease is seen in children also. With regard to the cause which produces it, very little is known; but it arises *immediately* from weakness of the kidneys. It must be borne in mind, that every excessive discharge of urine is not to be considered as diabetes, so great attention must be paid to the symptoms which I have described.

Treatment.—Physicians differ very much with regard to the treatment of this disease, and a great many remedies have been used, with various success. The disease is exceedingly dangerous, and you must not delay, but resort to medicine as soon as you are satisfied of the nature of the disease. If the pulse is full and harsh, and there are other signs of inflammation, and a fulness of the system, bleed moderately, and repeat the bleeding from time to time, taking a small quantity of blood at a time, until the bowels are natural. If the bowels are costive, keep them gently open with small doses of castor-oil, and laudanum, and clysters. Put cups over the kidneys (*see plates*), and blisters to the back, just above the fundament, or to the inside of the thighs, high up. As soon as the bowels are in a good state, give five grains of Dover's powder every four hours until the flow of urine is checked; or this: thirty drops of laudanum in a wineglassful of lime-water, three or four times a day. A great number of remedies have been employed in this disease, with various success, which you may try, if the treatment which I have recommended does not succeed.

Some of the preparations of iron, particularly the phosphate, magnesia, three or fours grains of the calcined, twice a day. In cases where the patient is much debilitated, five grains, gradually increased from day to day, of the carbonate of ammonia, three times a day. Peruvian bark, quinine, alum, nitric, sulphuric, muriatic acid, spirits of turpentine, tinct. cantharides, camphor, asafœtida, kino, &c.—(See table of medicines, for doses, &c.)   As a general rule, the patient must wear warm clothing, avoid exposure, take gentle exercise, drink no wine or spirits, except good brandy and water (weak), and take very light and wholesome food, such as is recommended for chronic inflammation of the mucous membrane of the bowels.—(Page 112.)

INSIPID DIABETES.

Under this head are comprised all of those complaints in which there is an excessive flow of urine, except the one just described as sweet diabetes.   In order, therefore, to distinguish them, you must pay great attention to the symptoms of each, as I have described them, particularly the color and appearance of the urine, remembering that every temporary profuse discharge of urine, is not to be regarded as diabetes ; as this may occur from drinking, changes of weather, particular drinks, teas, or vegetables, &c.   Again the urine of a person changes color frequently without disease ; sometimes it comes away very freely, and is nearly white, or it may be dark colored, with a muddy sediment, as you may have observed in the chamber, of a cold morning, &c.   But by attending carefully to all the symptoms which I have pointed out, you will find no difficulty in distinguishing the different kinds of diabetes, which is of great importance, as one kind is much more dangerous and difficult to cure than the other.

The next form of diabetes, is that in which a much greater quantity of what are called the earthy substances, or earthy phosphates, are formed in the urine.   For, I must here remark, that the urine is composed of a great many different substances mixed in certain proportions, when in a healthy state.   And whenever one substance is formed in greater quantity than another, it produces great distress.   In sweet diabetes, a quantity of sugar is formed, and this, of course, is taken away from the nourishment of the body ;

and so, also, when any of the other substances comes away in too great a quantity.

Symptoms of this form of diabetes.—An unnatural quantity of urine, sometimes very great, generally of a pale color, and sometimes white and altogether colorless. Sometimes, however, when the quantity is much greater than natural, the color is dingy or not transparent, and after it has stood some time, you will see a quantity of pale-colored grounds or sediment in the bottom of the chamber. It generally, too, smells bad after remaining a while. The patient generally suffers from indigestion, wind in the bowels, costiveness, or loose bowels, sick stomach, bad appetite, and great uneasiness after eating; a feeling of pain and uneasiness, or weakness, in the back or small of the back. The passages are sometimes black, or else the color of clay, or look like yeast. When the disease has far advanced, several other bad symptoms appear.

Treatment.—If the bowels are costive, give small doses of this mixture :—

  20 grains of rhubarb,
  40 grains of calcined magnesia,

well rubbed together, and put into a wineglassful of mint-water, or sugar and water; give half at a dose. When the bowels are opened, keep them open by giving two or three seidlitz powders a day. Give this, also :—

  2 drachms of the bicarbonate of soda,
  10 grains of sulphate of quinine,

rubbed up, and made into six powders; give one powder every two or three hours during the day ; and at night, give five grains of Dover's powder. Every other night, give this also :—

  4 grains of blue pill,
  2 grains of hippo,

made into one pill. Put a strengthening plaster, which you can get at any apothecary store, over the kidneys (see plates), or if you have not this, rub the place gently with turpentine or opodeldoc. After you have continued this treatment for some time, give this :—

  1 teaspoonful of nitric and muriatic acids,

in equal proportion, mixed together, and put into a tumbler of water. Let the patient suck through a quill, a wineglassful of this mixture every three or four hours during the day until the sediment in the urine changes color. After this, you may give quinine, or some of the preparations of iron. (See page 67.) With regard to the patient's food follow the directions for chronic inflammation of the mucous membrane of the bowels. (See page 112.)

There may be said to be two other forms of diabetes; one in which a greater quantity of what is called *urea* (one of the constituent principles of urine), is formed, than in any of the others. The last form, that in which one or more of the fluids which exist in the stomach and bowels, for the purpose of digesting the food, and nourishing the body, are brought away in the urine in quantity. These fluids are called chyle and albumen. But, as the symptoms which appear in these two forms, are by no means as conspicuous as those in the other two, and the complaints themselves by no means as dangerous, I must trust to your own judgment to treat them, after the remarks which I have made. In both of these last forms, the flow of urine is more or less increased, but the constitutional symptoms are, by no means, as conspicuous, important, or severe.

GRAVEL AND STONE IN THE BLADDER.

You must be careful not to confound this disease with diabetes, as you will see some of the symptoms much alike in both. By attending, however, to the following symptoms, you may easily distinguish them.

You will either see a *powder* of a reddish brown, or yellow color, sticking to the sides and bottom of the chamber after the urine has been allowed to stand awhile and cool, or small, irregular grains, like gravel, or coarse sand, which sink to the bottom of the chamber *immediately* as the urine is passed. Sometimes this powder and these grains unite and form a solid mass, of different sizes, which is called stone in the bladder.

Symptoms.—A frequent desire to pass water, a very little coming at a time, without giving relief: a heat and irritation about the neck of the bladder, and pain and uneasiness in the small of the back, about the kidneys. Wind-pains, and acid in the stomach and bowels, and symptoms of indigestion generally.

Treatment.—Attend particularly to the patient's food and bowels. He must eat nothing but the lightest and most wholesome food (see page 112), and keep the bowels open with these pills :—

    30 grains of blue pill,
     8 grains of aloes,

made into eight pills ; give one pill every other night, and if it does not operate, give two or three Seidlitz powders next morning. You may give this also—a teaspoonful of salæratus, in a wineglass of water. Soda water is good also ; and the patient should take a little of the infusion of gentian, or columbo root, three or four times a day. Sometimes you will see the urine in quantity, and of a pale color, and by examining it, when it has remained awhile, you will observe something like a thin, shining skin, all over the surface ; when this is the case, the urine is very apt to become offensive and putrid, and the symptoms, generally, are apt to be very distressing, as wind pains, sick stomach, costiveness, or loose bowels ; and the passages are sometimes black, whitish, or like yeast ; pain and weakness in the loins, &c., as in diabetes.

Treatment.—If the pulse is hard and full, and there are other symptoms of irritation and inflammation, cup the loins. —(See plates). Next put a compound galbanum plaster (commonly called a strengthening plaster), over the kidneys, and give opium in large doses, say from three to four grains at a dose, three times a day, until the patient is relieved. The patient must drink rain water, as hard water is very bad. Mercury, in no form must be given, unless in very small doses, with opium. If necessary, keep the bowels open with castor-oil, and injections; but if they are very loose, then give the mercury as directed.

When an attack of the gravel comes on (which you will know by the hard grains which I described), and there is much pain and distress, bleed, cup the kidneys, put the patient frequently into the warm bath, and give large doses of mercury, say eight or ten grains of calomel, with four grains of antimonial powder, at a dose, until the bowels are well emptied, and pay strict attention to the patient's food.

16

SUPPRESSION OF URINE FROM INFLAMMATION, OR PARALYSIS OF THE KIDNEYS, OR SOME MECHANICAL STOPPAGE, AS CALCULI, &c.

THIS disease must not be confounded with mere stoppage of the urine in the bladder, as it is very dangerous. There may be a complete, or only partial stoppage of the urine. The first is much more dangerous than the last.

Symptoms.—When the urine is not entirely suppressed, the patient passes a small quantity every now and then. He feels a dull, heavy weight about the hips, and sometimes pain and tenderness about the whole of the lower part of the belly, occasionally sickness at the stomach, or puking, &c. There is generally a good deal of fever. When the suppression is complete (that is to say, when he passes no water at all for some time), the patient can taste the urine in his mouth distinctly, and sometimes the whole body smells of urine. When the suppression occurs from paralysis of the kidneys, the painful symptoms seldom occur. From whatever cause, however, the suppression of urine occurs, if relief is not given, and the urine made to flow in about thirty-six hours, the head is apt to become affected. Other symptoms may appear, as a discharge of urinous fluids from the stomach, ears, &c. When the suppression is complete, the patient is apt to die in four or five days, or even sooner.

Treatment.—The treatment in this disease must depend upon the state of the kidneys, if it arises from inflammation of the kidneys.—(See inflammation of the kidneys, page 121.) Attend to the symptoms there described, and follow the directions. If the suppression is the consequence of paralysis of the kidneys, from a blow, fall, or any other accidental cause, or there is no active inflammation and pain, give spirits of turpentine and balsam copaiva, say twenty or thirty drops of either, every two hours during the day. And if the bowels are costive, give castor-oil and turpentine, until the bowels are well purged.—(See page 71.) If this treatment does not cause the urine to flow, put a large blister over the kidneys, and give doses of calomel or blue pill (see pages 31 and 20), until the patient is salivated, and give at the same time, diuretics freely.—(See from page 42 to 45.)

RETENTION OR STOPPAGE OF THE URINE IN THE BLADDER.

This may arise from inflammation of the bladder or surrounding parts, from clap, cantharides, turpentine, using the catheter carelessly, cold and damp feet, fevers, stoppage of the courses in women, falls and blows, and various other causes.   When the stoppage is from inflammation, you will observe the following

Symptoms.—A desire to make water frequently, attended with pain and distress; a severe burning pain, high up at the neck of the bladder, and just above the hair of the privates, and the parts between the privates and the fundament feel tender when they are pressed upon.   Fever, and sometimes sick stomach, and puking every now and then.   Great pain when you run a bougie or catheter up the penis.

Treatment.—If the patient is strong, bleed until he is sick at his stomach, then put several leeches between the privates and the fundament, and cup him just over the hair of the privates; or, if he is very hairy, shave some off very clean. When the leeches and cups have come away, he must sit down for some time, in a tub of warm water, up to the hips, to make the blood come away freely (that is, if he is not too weak from the bleeding), if so, wait awhile.   Next, give him several mild flaxseed clysters, warm (see page 70), until the bowels are well emptied; then let him take this:—

       8 grains of blue pill,
       4 grains of antimonial powder,

at one dose; if it does not operate in five hours, give a dose of castor-oil, or some mild purge.   The patient must, at the same time, drink this; a cupful of flaxseed tea, warm, with one or two grains of antimonial powder in it, every two hours. If this makes him sick at his stomach, lessen the quantity or stop awhile.   When he is relieved, and the water comes away, he must drink the flaxseed tea alone, and take three or four grains of the super-carbonate of soda, in a little water, three times a day, and keep on with the hip bath, and keep the bowels open with the clysters, and some mild purge every now and then.—(See page 30.)   If the water does not come away, put in a catheter.   Should the disease remain obstinate, see page 122, inflammation of the bladder, attend to the symptoms, and follow the directions given there.

Retention of urine may also be occasioned by chronic inflammation of the mucous membrane of the bladder, produced by clap badly treated, chronic diseases of the skin struck in, piles, gout and rheumatism transferred to the bladder, &c., and in this form is generally met with in old people.

Symptoms.—An uneasiness and tickling in the bladder, which extends down toward the privates. After some time, this feeling is changed to a constant gnawing pain, and there is difficulty in making water; and sometimes the water comes away of its own accord, and gives pain. The water has in it a quantity of mucus, like egg white, sometimes mixed with matter. This form of the disease is very serious, as the bladder is apt to be diseased.

Treatment.—(See page 124), chronic inflammation of the bladder—let the treatment be active or not, according to the symptoms, and follow the directions given there.

It may be produced by *paralysis*, or loss of power in the bladder; which may be brought on by various causes, as cold, and indisposition, looseness of the bowels (diarrhœa), piles dried up, fatigue, &c.

Symptoms.—The patient has to stand some time, and strain before he can make water, and when it does come, it flows gradually weaker, and in a small stream, and keeps him constantly straining, while the desire to make water is increased. No symptoms of inflammation, and the catheter can be passed in easily. This form is not dangerous, and is common in old persons.

Treatment.—Draw off the water with a silver catheter, or a bougie, every five or six hours. In introducing the catheter, be careful to turn the point upward, so that it may glide along the upper surface of the water passage, in the penis; and if you find it stop, do not push on, as there are folds of the membrane like little pockets, which you may tear, but draw it back a little, and push it gently again. Always push gently. Give this, also: 20 or 30 drops of the tincture of cantharides, in a little water, two or three times a day, until it produces painful symptoms, then stop, and rub the belly with it. If this does no good, put a blister just above the hair of the privates; and give spirits of turpentine (see page 45), or balsam copaiva (see page 50). Use clysters of cold water, &c.

The stoppage may occur suddenly, and the patient feel a great desire, and make frequent attempts to pass his urine without being able to pass more than a few drops, and those with great pain. In this case, the stoppage is caused by a spasmodic contraction and closure of some part of the urethra, or water-passage. There is a cutting pain in the bladder, and a feeling of bearing down, such as women in labor feel. The patient generally feels a tenderness from the orifice of the penis, throughout, and is frequently troubled with erections of the penis. The pain is greater just after the last few drops of water come away, and the patient feels a spasm about the place between the privates and the fundament (called the perinæum). In this variety, the pain is not continued, and the disease frequently terminates with a free discharge of urine. No fever, pulse small, difficulty of passing a catheter, very great. Spasmodic retention of urine may also occur as a consequence of inflammation of the urinary organs, and may arise from cold, damp feet, clap, stimulating injections, distressing or exciting emotions of the mind, &c. It is not, in general, very obstinate or dangerous, unless neglected, or inflammation comes on.

Treatment.—Put the patient into a warm bath, and give him twenty drops of the tincture of the muriate of iron, every fifteen minutes, unless there is much inflammation, or you suspect that the patient has a stricture. Give anodyne clysters, also.—(See page 70.) If these fail to bring away the water, and the patient is distressed, put in a catheter; but, if you find the catheter stopped, or stick in the passage as if it was grasped by something, stop and rub the place between the privates and the fundament with the fingers of your other hand, but do not jerk. Lastly, if these fail, give large doses of opium (see page 15), or these pills :—

     5 grains of opium,
    40 grains of gum asafœtida,
     5 grains of hippo,

rubbed up with a few drops of the oil of peppermint, and made into twelve pills; give one pill every hour, until the patient is relieved.

Retention of urine may occur from stricture, and requires very prompt treatment. When this happens, bleed immediately from the arms, cup the loins, and put several leeches about the fundament, and near by. Then put the patient into a warm bath, and give him injections of warm water, with a little sweet oil, frequently. After the bowels have been

16*

well emptied in this way, give anodyne clysters (see page 70),
and five grains of Dover's powder every three hours ; putting
the patient into the warm bath every now and then, and giving
him to drink freely of such drinks as flaxseed tea, warm, and
such as are mentioned under the head of diluents (page 39).
Should these means fail, introduce a small bougie, with great
care, if possible. If the patient is a female, use the female
catheter.

Lastly, retention of urine may occur from some obstruction
of the water-passage, or neck of the bladder, from a calculus,
(stone), clotted blood, tumors, &c., and in women from pregnancy, the heavy womb pressing on the water-passage. In
every case, the treatment must depend on the cause of the
stoppage. Follow the directions which I have given, and
use your judgment.

STRANGURY, OR DIFFICULTY AND PAIN IN MAKING WATER.

Symptoms.—Water passed slowly, frequently, with pain,
and a straining about the fundament, particularly just as the
last drops comes away; an uneasy feeling high up in the
bladder, and a burning or cutting pain in the water-passage.
This complaint is common and very distressing, and may be
brought on by the following causes, as taking cantharides,
blisters near the bladder, piles becoming inflamed, drinking,
eating too much, and unwholesome food, excessive venereal
indulgence, suppressed courses in women, calculi, gravel, and
stone in the bladder, gout, rheumatism, from worms in children, fevers, clap-injections, and some other causes.

Treatment.—The treatment of this complaint must depend
upon the cause which produces it. If it arises from accidental irritation, as clap, or recent inflammation, open the
bowels with some mild purge, as castor-oil, or Epsom salts,
give the patient an anodyne clyster, put him to bed, and let
him drink freely of warm flaxseed tea, and diluent drinks.—
(See page 39.) If these do not relieve, put leeches to the
privates and the fundament ; let the patient sit frequently and
for some time, in a large tub of warm water, and give a table-

spoonful of spirits of nitre in a pint of tea ; or, if necessary, introduce a catheter carefully. Use this same treatment when it arises from cantharides. Sometimes it occurs in females from the whites ; when this is the case, take two grains of lunar caustic, dissolve them in a small wineglass of water ; then take five or six grains of opium, and dissolve it in the same quantity of hot water, strain it clear ; mix the two mixtures together, and syringe with this three times a day. Use a *female syringe*, to be had at any apothecary store. To cure the whites, use this at the same time ; five grains of white vitriol, or fifteen grains of alum, dissolved in a large wineglass of warm water ; syringe with this carefully, frequently, during the day. When the complaint is brought on by gravel, stone, or sediment in the urine, see these diseases (pages 180 and 181), and follow the treatment there directed. When it arises from the piles, see pages 162 and 163, and attend to the directions given there. When it occur in nervous and hysterical women, who are liable to it, and feel great pain in the bladder, at times, just after making water, give this :—

    4 grains of Dover's powder,
    2 grains of camphor,

rubbed up, and made into one powder ; to be taken three or four times a day. When it occurs in infants, from teething, they generally scream when making water. In such cases, open the bowels with rhubarb, or castor-oil (see page 33), and give this :—

    1 grain of calomel,
    2 grains of hippo,

rubbed up, and made into five or six powders ; give one powder twice or three times a day, and in the evening, two or three drops of laudanum, in a little warm flaxseed tea.

    This complaint is seen also in old people, and is generally caused by some disorder of the bladder ; in these cases, let a physician examine carefully, and find out the cause.

INABILITY TO RETAIN THE URINE — IT COMING
AWAY INVOLUNTARILY, BY DROPS, OR ALL AT
ONCE.

THIS complaint may arise from various causes, as injuries
of the spine from falls or blows, stone and gravel in the bladder or kidneys, paralysis of the bladder, as in old people, from
injuries of the brain, from difficult labor in women, tumors
about the bladder, pregnancy. It is seen in nervous and
hysterical persons, and in children, and may occur from
many other causes.

Treatment.—The treatment of this complaint must depend
on the cause which produces it. As a general rule, always
examine the water, to see if there is any sediment, or gravel
in it, particularly in children, or get a physician to examine
it. If you find sediment, or gravel, see pages 180 and 181,
for directions. When. the complaint seems to arise from
paralysis or weakness of the bladder, you may adopt the following treatment, according to circumstances : 20 grains of
alum, in a little mucilage of gum arabic, every four or five
hours during the day, for a grown person; or 15 drops of
the tincture of cantharides, three or four times a day, in a
little water, until the patient feels a difficulty and pain in
making water. The dose of this last medicine may be increased to twenty, twenty-five, or thirty drops at a dose, or
even more, every day. - Use, at the same time, bathing with
cold water, frequently repeated ; injections of cold water up
the fundament, and cold water poured, from a height, on the
belly, over the bladder, just above the privates. — (See
plates.)

If these do not succeed, put blisters to the back, just above
the fundament, or cup the place between the fundament and
the privates, called the perinœum. When it occurs in nervous persons, give anodyne clysters (see page 70), Dover's
powders, some of the preparations of iron and zinc, uva
ursi.—(See pages 36, 45, and 67.) When in females from
the whites, see page 149, and follow the directions there
given. When from piles, or ascarides, see pages 162 and
171.

GONORRHŒA, OR CLAP, ALSO CALLED THE RUNNING.

Symptoms.—About three or four days, sometimes two days, and sometimes eight or ten days, after a person has been with a female of bad character, he will feel a disagreeable itching about the orifice of the water-passage, at the extremity of the privates. When this itching has lasted about a day, the mouth of the water-passage will appear inflamed and swollen, and a whitish or yellowish matter, will ooze out of it. After this the stinging and itching increase, and when the person makes water, it burns or scalds very much. The disease soon becomes worse, and the patient is apt to feel very painful erections of his yard, particularly after going to bed, called chordee. When this disease occurs in women, they do not feel the same inconvenience as men, and they may even have it very bad, without suffering much pain. Sometimes, however, they feel a severe scalding, on making water, and there is a great deal of inflammation about their privates, which causes great soreness and pain, and considerable running, which, at times, gets on the inside of the thighs, and causes pimples, &c.

Treatment.—Whether the patient is a man or woman, at the commencement of the disease, give every day, for three or four days, a dose of Epsom salts, with half a grain of tartar emetic in each dose. At the same time, the patient must drink freely of warm flaxseed tea, all day, each pint of the flaxseed tea having in it, eight or ten grains of saltpetre, or a tablespoonful of spirits of nitre. Bathe the privates, also, frequently in warm water, or put warm, soft poultices to them. If the chordee is troublesome, take one grain of opium, with eight grains of camphor, just before you go to bed. Sometimes bleeding takes place from the water-passage ; when this occurs, do not attempt to stop it, unless it is very great, as it generally relieves the inflammation. But, if it becomes profuse, just seize the yard with one hand, and squeeze it for 20 or 30 minutes, when it will stop. The patient must remain quiet, not ride on horseback, walk much, or drink any wine or spirits, nor eat rich or salt food. When you have continued this treatment about three or four days, and the inflammation is somewhat subdued, give this :—

½ wineglassful of balsam copaiva,
1 tablespoonful of spirits of nitre,
2 teaspoonfuls of laudanum,
30 grains of gum arabic (powder),

dissolved in a wineglass of hot water.   Mix and shake well.
Give a teaspoonful of this mixture four or five times a day.
When the patient can not take balsam in this way, give the
copaiva capsules, beginning with three a day, and increasing
to six a day.   If the disease is of long standing, give this :—

½ wineglassful of balsam copaiva,
½   do.   tincture of cubebs,
1 tablespoonful spirits of nitre,
1 teaspoonful laudanum,
1 teaspoonful of powdered gum arabic,

in a tumblerful of warm water, sweetened with white sugar.
Mix and shake well, and give a tablespoonful 4 or 5 times a day.

After the disease has lasted sometime, and the pain, soreness and inflammation seem to have subsided, if the running
is obstinate, and becomes white, like cream, or ropy and
stringy, give this :—

3 teaspoonfuls of tincture of cubebs,
1 teaspoonful of spirits of turpentine,

in a little water, three or four times a day, or this :—

20 to 25 drops of tincture of cantharides,

increasing the dose daily, until the patient feels pain and difficulty in making water, then stop awhile.—(See page 184.)
If these fail, try injections, as follows :—

1 grain of the sulphate of zinc,

dissolved in a wineglass of water; syringe this carefully up
the penis.   You will find it necessary to change the injection
every now and then, another is :—

1 drop of sulphuric acid,
In a wineglass of water.

These may be increased in strength gradually.   Another is :—

6 or 8 drops of pyroligneous acid,
Or, 4 drops of kreosote water,

in a large wineglass of water.   There are several other kinds
of injections.   A gleet is sometimes very obstinate, and will
resist almost every remedy.   When this is the case, smear a
bougie with mercurial ointment, and push it some distance
up the penis.   This, however, must not be done if there is
tenderness and inflammation.   Some persons get rid of this
disease more easily, and in a shorter time than others.

THE VENEREAL DISEASE—THE SIMPLE VENEREAL ULCER.

Symptoms.—From three to five, or even eight days, after connexion with a female of bad character, you will feel an itching generally about the inner part of the foreskin of your yard, and see a redness about the place, and a short time afterward, a small pimple or pustule, surrounded by a red edge or margin. This pimple, in a few days, is changed into a thin crust, with matter under it, and becomes quite painful. By degrees the scab becomes larger, of a round or triangular shape, and of a yellowish or dark-brown color. The scab now soon falls off, and leaves an ulcer, or sore, of an oval or round shape, of a reddish or dirty-yellow color, glossy or shining, and having a narrow red circle of inflammation around it. After this, the sore begins to fill up from the bottom, until it is higher than the surface of the skin around, of a healthy color, smooth, of a somewhat spongy or fungous appearance, and the bottom and edge of a darker-red color than the rest of the sore. The sore is at its greatest height about the fourteenth or fifteenth day, and about this time the ulceration and inflammation cease or have ceased.

The foreskin, in this disease, is apt to become inflamed and to close over the head of the yard, preventing the urine from coming away, and causing what is called *phimosis.* A discharge like clap also very frequently comes on.

This disease is produced by the matter of clap, or unclean and vitiated matter, in the organs of the female, and is not classed among those called syphilis or pox, although, like them, it is sometimes followed by secondary or constitutional symptoms, which are as follows:—

Slight fever and headache, pains in the joints, and sometimes in the chest; after this an eruption of pale-red or deep-crimson spots or pimples, which become of a paler or copper color, and generally scale off when they are about to disappear, and they come about five weeks, or even three or four months, after the commencement of the disease. The throat and tonsils also become swollen, but not ulcerated, as in true syphilis.

Treatment.—From the commencement of the disease, the patient must keep quiet; keep the bowels open with gentle

medicines, and take very light food.   If there is much inflammation and irritation of the system, bleed and keep him
in bed.   If the skin closes over the yard, and there is pain,
inflammation, and swelling there, put warm soft poultices to
the place (see page 69), and observe if matter is forming under the string of the yard : if so, you must get a physician to
let it out.   When there is not much irritation, put on warm,
soft, light poultices (taking care not to let them get hard)
until the scab comes off the pimple—that is, if the pimple is
on the outside of the yard; but when it is on the inside of
the foreskin, keep a piece of linen rag, wet with weak lead-
water, between the skin and the head of the yard.   After
the scab has dropped off, you may use this as a wash to the
sore :—

6 grains of corrosive sublimate,
In 4 wineglasses of lime-water ;

wet a rag, and wash the sore gently four or five times a day
with it.

THE SUPERFICIAL VENEREAL ULCER, OR PUSTULE, WITH WELL-MARKED AND RAISED EDGES.

Symptoms.—A small pimple or pustule, generally on the
outside of the foreskin, or the skin of the yard itself; sometimes on the forepart of the stone-bag.   Sometimes it is seen
all around the front edge of the foreskin, and when it heals,
leaves a lasting phimosis.   The pimple soon breaks after it
is formed, and leaves a crust, beneath which the skin breaks
or ulcerates, and makes a sore or ulcer, of a round or oval
shape.   After the crust comes off, an ulcer is left, of a reddish-brown color, with raised and distinct edges, and having
its surface on a level with, or somewhat raised above the
level of the skin around.   There is no hardness around the
ulcer, not much pain, and its size varies from that of a pea
to a ten-cent piece ; but if neglected, or badly managed, it is
apt to spread and become much larger.   This ulcer generally takes some time to heal, but does not spread.   In this
form of the disease, secondary or constitutional symptoms
generally or always come on at various periods from the commencement of the disease, which are as follows : an eruption

on the skin of various parts of the body, of pimples or pustules. These pimples or pustules do not come out all at once, or run their course at the same time; but while some are just forming, others are scabbing. You will see also small ulcers, or sores, from which the scabs have already fallen, between these pustules, and the skin discolored in spots and patches, showing where the ulcers have been and healed up. The throat and tonsils also are very apt to become inflamed and ulcerated, and the patient apt to feel pains like those of acute rheumatism.

Treatment.—If the irritation of the system is great, bleed, purge out the bowels well, and give such medicines as are directed under the head of Diaphoretics (see pages 35 and 36) Nitre, and Antimonials, and put soft warm poultices to the sores, if there is much inflammation (see page 69). If there is not much pain and inflammation, wash the ulcers with this, four or five times a day:—

4 grains of the white vitriol (sulphate of zinc),
Or sugar of lead,

dissolved in a wineglass of water. The use of calomel or mercury, in any form, is generally considered wrong in this disease.

THE HARD-SLOUGHING VENEREAL ULCER.

Symptoms.—This species of venereal ulcer or sore is seen frequently where the foreskin folds or doubles, at the neck of the yard, just behind the ridge of the head, called the ● crown of the glans of the penis or yard. It is attended with much inflammation and pain about the sore, and general bad health. The sore is very apt to slough, as it is called, which is a destruction or rotting of the flesh around it, and generally forms a deep ulcer or hole between the skin and body of the yard. The ulcer is hard, like cartilage or gristle, at the bottom, unless it is on the head of the yard. The sore is frequently seen also on the inside of the foreskin, covered with a dark, liver-colored stuff, like decayed flesh, which soon falls off; and this goes on until the ulcer becomes deep, but it does not spread much. Mortification of the parts

17

around the sore, is very apt to occur, sometimes to a considerable extent, and in a very short time. After the sores are healed, the spots where they have been, remain hard, and if they are rubbed or bruised, or not kept clean, are apt to break out again.

This form of the disease is frequently followed by constitutional symptoms, which appear at times so soon, that they may be said almost to attend the disease. They are as follows:

Secondary Symptoms.—A feeling of weariness and sickness generally, restlessness at night, pale countenance, and dull, drooping eyes, for some days. Sometimes a soreness of the chest and breast, some difficulty of breathing, tenderness of the scalp, and headache at night; and sometimes considerable fever. These symptoms, or some of them, usually last for several days, and then pimples, like warts, spots, or pustules, something like small-pox, come out, which quickly change into sores, with thick scabs, and spread around at the same time that they are healing in the middle. Pains of the joints, knees, and wrists, swelling of the testicles, ulcerations, destroying the soft bones of the nose, in the throat, destroying the palate and tonsils, which, as they increase, are apt to reduce the patient to a state like consumption.

Treatment.—If there is much irritation of the system, pain and swelling about the foreskin, great uneasiness, heat and dryness of the skin, bleed immediately and put the patient to bed; purge out the bowels well, and give this:—

    1 grain of tartar emetic, or,
    2 teaspoonfuls of antimonial wine,

in a large tumbler of water; give a tablespoonful every hour. Give this internally:—

    4 grains of the sulphate of morphine,
    40 grains of blue pill,

rubbed up, and made into eight pills; give one pill in the morning, and another in the evening. Continue these until the gums are a little sore, then stop awhile. Or the calomel and opium pills.—(See page 71.) Give one in the morning, midday, and evening. If the patient becomes very weak, give him quinine. Put warm soft poultices to the sores until the decayed flesh separates (see page 69), and then wash and dress the sores with this:—

    8 grains of calomel,
    In a wineglass of lime water.

THE SOFT SLOUGHING VENEREAL ULCER, OR THE PHAGEDENIC ULCER.

Symptoms.—This ulcer is generally seen on the head or glans of the yard, near the foreskin. The foreskin is apt to slough or rot and fall off, and frequently the whole head of the yard. When the head of the yard has dropped off, the sore begins to heal. Sometimes, also, but not often, the ulcer goes on sloughing, until the whole yard slowly rots and drops off. The ulcer, when it first makes its appearance, is of an irregular shape or appearance, as if eaten out by a worm, or corroded by some destructive caustic; but has *no hardness* around it, as in the other form just described. It sometimes spreads rapidly, sometimes slowly.

Treatment.—If possible, remove the patient to a pure air, (that of Aiken is excellent). But if there is much inflammation, bleed immediately, and put the patient to bed; put warm soft poultices (flaxseed poultices are good), to the whole yard.—(See page 69.) Wash the sore frequently with warm water and castile soap. Let the patient take this:—

    1 pint of flaxseed tea, warm,
    1 tablespoonful of antimonial wine;

mix and give a small wineglassful every hour, or even oftener, so as to keep the patient sick at his stomach. After the inflammation has been subdued, and the sloughing checked, if the ulceration becomes obstinate, as sometimes happens, healing in one place, and spreading in another, wash the sore with this, four or five times a day:—

    2 grains of the nitrate of silver,
    In a wineglass of water.

If this does no good, try the wash, page 192, or that on page 194. If the ulcer is very ragged, you may cut away the diseased or ragged part, carefully, with a sharp lancet or knife, and encourage the piece to bleed with warm water.

Physicians generally agree that the use of mercury in this form, is decidedly injurious. Keep the bowels gently open, and if the patient is restless, give small doses of opium.—(See page 29.)

SYPHILIS, OR GENUINE POX.

THE CHANCRE.—This may be distinguished by the following *Symptoms.*—An ulcer of a round shape, as if dug out, or scooped out of the flesh, its inside surface perfectly smooth, with matter sticking to it, and the edges and bottom of the ulcer hard, like cartilage or gristle. This cartilaginous hardness is immediately around the ulcer, and does not extend any distance, but terminates suddenly, as you will observe, if you pinch up the ulcer between your fingers. This ulcer generally makes its appearance somewhere on the head or glans of the yard; but it is also seen on the body or shaft of the yard, and in this case has a somewhat different appearance, being of a dark liver color, with none, or very little, cartilaginous hardness around it, and having none of that scooped or dug-out appearance about it. Remember this—a true chancre is always indolent or sluggish in its nature, and slow in its progress. You must not, however, suppose that every sore or ulcer which is found on the head of the yard, and has hard cartilaginous edges, is pox.

The constitutional, or secondary symptoms of the Chancre.—These consist of spots on the skin, slightly raised, and covered with hard thin, whitish scales, which easily drop off, and leave smooth, shining marks, of a copper color. Sometimes these spots cluster together, and form patches of an irregular shape, copper color, and having portions of loose scales hanging to them. These spots are generally seen on the forehead, neck, breast, belly, arms, and legs. You will sometimes, also, observe dry scales in the palms of the hands, and soles of the feet, which are easily broken up, and when they drop off, leave the place where they have been, thick and hard, and of a dark, dingy color.

When the eruption comes out on the stone bag, between the cheeks of the bomb, under the arms, or in any concealed place, where the skin touches or rubs, the spots are not hard and scaly, but raised, soft and clammy, with a whitish matter oozing from their surface.

The dry, scaly spots on the body, if not attended to when they first appear, are apt to form scabs or crusts, with matter under them, and where they fall off, to leave ulcers.

These eruptions are frequently seen upon the mouth and throat. After some time, also, the throat becomes ulcerated, and the ulcers, which are generally on the tonsils, look like those first seen on the yard, not being preceded or surrounded by much inflammation. The covering of the bones, also, and the bones themselves, near the skin, as the skull, breast-bone, and collar-bone, are apt to become affected, and enlarge or swell, without much pain, or discoloring of the skin, until the disease is much advanced. These risings on the bones are called nodes.

Treatment of the Chancre.—Wash the ulcer frequently, and dress it with a little simple ointment or lint.—(See page 69.) Then give this:—

    24 grains of calomel,
     3 grains of gum opium (powdered),
made into twelve pills; give one pill morning, noon, and night, until the gums are sore. Or this:—

    48 grains of blue-pill,
     3 grains of the sulphate of morphine,
rubbed up and made into twelve pills; give them in the same way, until the gums are sore. As soon as the gums are sore, touch the edges of the chancre all round with lunar caustic, and wash it, several times a day, with the wash (page 195). The gums must be kept sore (but avoid producing severe salivation) for six weeks or two months, and continue this treatment during this time. The patient must wear warm clothing, avoid exposure, drink no spirits, eat nothing but light food, and keep quiet.

After this treatment has been continued for three months (as a general rule), and the patient seems to be no better, salivate him with this:—

    10 grains of calomel,
made into one powder, and given, every night and morning, until he is decidedly salivated; then purge out his bowels with a full dose of Epsom salts (see page 32), if the calomel has not purged him too severely.

As a general rule, while you are giving medicine for the cure of this disease, you may give this, as a drink; a good handful of sarsaparilla root, broken up, and a large table-spoonful of the dry leaves of queen's delight; put these into a pot with a quart of water, and a teacupful of molasses. Boil them fifteen minutes, and then throw in a teaspoonful of rhubarb, powdered. Cover the pot, and let it boil slowly for half an hour, or until about a half-pint, or more, of the

17*

water has boiled away. Then take it off, put the mixture into bottles, well corked. Give a wineglassful three or four times a day, or, in obstinate cases, oftener.

Should this treatment which I have recommended, not succeed, you must apply to a physician. There are many remedies which I could mention, such as Fowler's solution of arsenic, ioduret of mercury, acetate of copper (or verdigris), carbonate of ammonia, and sulphate of zinc (or white vitriol). All of these have been frequently used, but according to my opinion and experience, some cases are benefited by one medicine, and other cases by others, and the directions that I have given, are the safest to follow, as a general rule. Some physicians give no mercury at all.

BUBOES.

Whenever you see a rising or swelling, of a long shape, in the crease between the thigh and the belly, you may suspect it to be a bubo. You must be careful, however, not to mistake a femoral hernia, or rupture, for one. They are easily distinguished, for if you make the patient lie on his back and put his feet up against the wall, if it is a rupture, the gut will either go up into the belly itself, and the rising disappear, or you can easily push it up with your fingers; and you are apt to hear a gurgling sound, as the gut is going back. The gut, however, may have stuck to the parts around, and so can not be pushed back, and the swelling will remain. In this case, the swelling will begin on the belly and run across the crease, on to the thighs. But a bubo generally lies in the crease, beginning above and running down toward the stone-bag. A bubo also feels either hard and lumpy, or is very painful and inflamed, while a rupture is puffy.

Buboes are of two kinds: sympathetic buboes, which are seen in clap, are hard, lumpy, and generally not painful, and do not require any treatment. Those which are seen in syphilis, or pox, may be known by the following signs :—

Symptoms.—A rising in the groin, on one or both sides, either very painful, with a hard, full and quick pulse, and a general irritation of the whole system, or, with no pain, hard, and a general weakness or debility of the system.

If the bubo is inflamed and of the former kind, bleed the patient, and put leeches all around the bubo, and when these drop off, put on large, warm, light poultices.—(See page 69.) If the bubo comes to a head, like a bile, and does not break, and the skin is smooth, shining, and thin, showing matter in it, open it with a lancet, and keep it running with warm poultices. Rub the inner part of the thighs with mercurial ointment, once or twice a day; purge out the patient well with Epsom salts, and let him drink this—1 pint of flaxseed tea, kept warm, with 1 or 2 grains of tartar emetic in it, or a good tablespoonful of antimonial wine. Give a wineglassful of this mixture every two or three hours, so as to keep the patient sick at his stomach. Continue this treatment for two or three days, until the symptoms of inflammation disappear. Keep the patient in bed, on very simple and light food, and when the poultices are stopped, dress the bubo with rags wet with lead-water.

If the bubo, on the contrary, is indolent, and remains without coming to a head, or scattering, put blisters on it. As soon as one comes off, and dries up, put on another. If the blisters bring the bubo to a head, and you see matter in it, open it with a lancet, and put on warm, soft, light poultices, to keep it running. Sometimes after a bubo has burst, or been opened, the place remains soft and unhealthy, and discharges a watery stuff. When this happens, use this;

5 grains of corrosive sublimate, dissolved in
8 large wineglasses of lime-water.

Squirt some of this into the bubo, with a small syringe, three or four times a day, and put on it warm, soft poultices, each mixed with two or three teaspoonfuls of Peruvian bark powder. If the patient is weak and much debilitated by the disease, give one grain of opium, or a quarter of a grain of sulphate of morphine, every night.

Keep the patient quiet, the bowels open, and give gentle sweats. Sometimes the opening in the bubo will not heal, and has fungous, projecting edges, like proud flesh; in such cases, a physician must cut them off with a knife or lancet.

MIDWIFERY.

How to put a woman to bed and deliver her.—As soon as the labor pains come on, let the woman go to bed. Next, when you wish to fix her for delivery, bring her down to the foot of the bed, draw up her knees until the heels touch the breech; then draw the knees wide apart, so as to open the thighs well, and support the knees by putting a pillow, or pillows, under each of them, on the outside, so as to leave the space between the woman's legs clear. Fold up a sheet or blanket four times, and put it under her rump, for the waters, &c. Put a pillow under the small of her back, and one under her head, if she wishes.

Get everything now ready. Two or three needlefuls of white Osnaburg thread, well waxed; a tub of warm water, soft soap (castile is the best), and a sharp pair of scissors. Take a piece of soft linen rag, about eight inches square, cut a hole in the middle of it, about the size of a quarter of a dollar, and smear one side of the rag with fresh hog's lard, or mutton suet, for the navel-string.

When the waters have come away, if the pains do not come on strong in a quarter of an hour, or so (as a general rule), put your hand into cold water, and put it on the woman's belly above the hair of the privates, to make the womb contract, and you may even rub the belly gently, or squeeze it a little. If the pains slacken, the woman may change her position for a while, or even get up and walk about the room, until the pains come on strong enough. Then put her back in the same position. When the child's head shows, it is always a safe plan (particularly with women in their first confinement), for the midwife, or physician, to press the back of the hand (that part between the thumb and first finger of the right hand), up against that part of the woman which is between the hole of her fundament and the bottom corner of her privates, where the slit begins. Because, the privates here are very thin, and the child's head coming very suddenly against it, or through it, before it has had time to stretch, is apt to tear it. Besides, some women have a short slit and a deep pit or bag here inside; and when the child's head slips down into this, it requires to be pressed up, that it may come through the slit of the woman.

As soon as the child is born, tie the navel-string strongly

about four inches from the child's belly, with one thread, and about three quarters of an inch from this, tie the navel-string again, then cut between the two threads. You may now bring the woman's knees together, and let her lie comfortably, until the next strong pain, which brings the after-birth. If the pains do not come on in a quarter or half an hour or so, put your cold hand on her belly, and do as I directed before.

When the after-birth comes down so that you can see it, or feel it with your fingers, take hold of the cord with your left hand, very gently, and pass your right hand gently up until you can grasp the after-birth. Then, if a good pain comes on, or the woman bears down well, draw the cord very gently and slowly until the whole of the after-birth comes away. Be careful not to pull hard or to be on a hurry, and see that you take away all the bags of the waters (or membranes), along with the after-birth (or placenta).

As soon as the after-birth has come away, the doctor or midwife should put their hand on the woman's belly, just above the the privates, and, by grasping it and pressing the fingers down gently, feel if the womb has contracted. If the womb has contracted, you will feel a hard ball under your hand. You can then go away; but unless you feel this ball, you should remain; because the womb is apt to bleed inside, and the mouth being shut up, it will bleed until it gets so full that it can not hold more blood, and the mouth of the womb will suddenly open, and the blood gush out in such quantities as to kill the woman suddenly, sometimes even while she is sleeping quietly.

No doctor or midwife ought then to leave the room or let the woman go to sleep, until they have felt and satisfied themselves that the womb has contracted into a hard ball; then there is not much danger of its bleeding too much.

Just before a woman is confined, give her a dose of castor-oil, or an injection; it is apt to give her an easier time. And after she is confined, she must be kept quiet and still in bed, for several days. Because, if she gets up or exerts herself to rise, and sit up in the bed, she is apt to produce falling of the womb; and if she talks much, to have fever.

. After confinement, put a swathe, or band, around the woman's belly, not too tight.

Dressing the Child.—As soon as the child's navel-string is cut, wash it carefully all over, head and all, in blood-warm water and soap (castile soap if you have it, if not, any other kind). I have seen it stated in a certain book of medicine, that "it is wrong to wash the child, and that it should be dressed just as it comes from the mother." Such a practice I think not only *filthy*, but positively injurious to the child; because, the sticky matter which covers the child, if it become dry and hard under the arms, and other tender parts, is very apt to produce sores. And I can assure the reader, that I have had every child that I ever attended, washed, and not one was injured.

Now wipe the child carefully, taking care not to rub or jerk the navel-string, for it is n t to become dry and stick to the towel; and es. a good many cases of locked-jaw are bro read. handling the navel-string too roughly. Cut o. as of the thread, then push the navel-string carefully through the hole in the rag, which I have directed, letting the *dry* side lay flat on the child's belly, the greased side up; now turn the navel-string down on the rag, pointing upward toward the child's chest, and fold the lower part of the rag over it, fold the two sides of the rag again over this, and put a loose, light bandage over, all around the child's belly. Now dress it, and as soon as you can put it to the mother's breast, let it nurse.

A black stuff always comes away from the child for some little time after it is born (called the *meconium*). The mother's milk is generally sufficient to bring this away. But if it does not come away freely, give the child a teaspoonful of sweet-oil, or best castor-oil. If a child is still-born, rub the body and limbs with some spirit, and put vinegar, burnt feathers, or even hartshorn to the nose. I have sometimes, in obstinate cases, even poured hartshorn up the child's nose, and saved it.

SURGERY.

How to cure a Cut.—Wipe the blood off dry, and bring the edges of the cut together as soon as possible, with your fingers, then cover the cut with a piece of adhesive strap, the yellow side held over a shovel of hot coals. Leave a little corner of the cut uncovered, for the matter to ooze out, always the lowest corner, so that the matter will not run on the strap.

If the cut has been left open, however, and is much inflamed, put warm poultices, until the inflammation is reduced, and then put on the straps. Put on fresh straps about every two days (unless the wound runs much, then every day), taking care to leave one old strap on until you put on a fresh one. Always wash the cut clean with water and castile soap, and wipe it dry or the straps will not stick.

Boils.—Bring the boil to a head, by using warm, soft poultices (see page 69), and if it does not burst itself, open it with a lancet. Be careful not to open it before it comes to a head.

Gunshot Wounds.—If no physician can be had, keep the wound constantly clean, by washing it with castile soap and warm water; and keep on it constantly, warm, soft, light poultices, changing them and putting on fresh ones frequently. Never let the poultice get hard or cold. A gunshot wound seldom bleeds much, unless some large blood-vessel is cut. But it sloughs and becomes very offensive, until all the flesh destroyed by the shot, or ball, rots and falls off; then it begins to heal. When it begins to heal, treat it like other wounds, dressing it with soft linen rags, smeared with simple ointment.—(See page 69.)

Burns and Scalds.—These are the most unmanageable kind of injuries, and when bad, sometimes defy all treatment. As a general rule, keep the burnt or scalded places constantly covered with soft rags, smeared with fresh hog's lard, or wet with lead-water. Be careful not to let two surfaces of the skin touch, or they may stick, and when burns or scalds are near joints, keep the limb stretched, or it is apt to draw up and grow so.

Carbuncle.—This is generally seen on the back, and looks like a large boil, is very painful and hard to come to a head. It must be cut open, and all the diseased stuff squeezed out, or pulled out with a pair of dressing forceps, then washed out clean, and the hole filled up with lint, greased with simple ointment. (See page 69.) This must be pulled out every morning, and fresh lint put in. When the wound is clean and disposed to heal, put poultices on it, and treat it as a boil or other wound.

Broken Bones.—If no doctor can be had, put the limb straight and try and set it. You can generally tell when a bone is straight by looking at the other limb, and passing your finger along the bone. Keep the limb quiet and straight, by putting on splints of pasteboard wet and moulded to the shape of the limb. Over these put light wooden splints, but be careful not to bandage a broken limb tight, for it swells and becomes very painful. When the bone is knitting, you will see a lump. Take great care that the patient does not break the bone again, for it is very weak just after it has knit. A bone generally knits in about six weeks, but the bandages ought to be kept on sometime after. It is useless to say anything about dislocations and other surgical cases, for they require a physician, and no person should attempt to manage them without a physician, and, of course, the patient must take his chance, if one can not be had.

How to pull a Tooth.—Take the instrument called the key instrument; fix the claw so that the bolster will always press on the gum inside the jaw, next to the tongue. Cut the gum close to and all around the tooth, down to the bone, with a gum lancet. Wrap a piece of rag around the bolster, so as not to bruise the gum. Let the patient sit down in a chair, and throw his head back, and open his mouth wide. Now for the upper jaw stand behind him, for the lower, before him (as a general rule). When the bolster of the instrument touches the gum, put the claw over the tooth, and let the sharp points pass in between the gum of the opposite side and the neck of the tooth. Try your instrument by turning the handle a little, to see if it is firmly fixed. If so, turn steadily, but not with too much force, always inward toward the tongue, the bolster kept steady on the gum, and the tooth will come out. If the tooth is hard to come, try another claw, but do not force.

How to bleed.—Let the patient sit up in the bed, or in a chair; make the arm which you are going to bleed from bare. Tie a piece of list or broad tape, by winding it three or four times around the arm, just above the elbow joint, moderately tight, but not so tight as to stop the pulse of that arm. Next, feel the vein in the hollow of the elbow, below the bandage, to try if it has swelled out, and feels tight, grasp the arm with your left hand, and keep your thumb pressed upon the vein, just below where you are going to stick it. Next, hold your lancet in your right hand, and let the point touch the middle of the vein, just above the thumb which is on it. Now push it firmly and steadily into the vein; taking care not to move your thumb, and not to let the point of the lancet go too straight or too deep down, for you may cut through the other side of the vein; but cut from you upward. A small cut just allowing the point of the lancet to go into the vein is generally sufficient. As soon as you take off your thumb, the blood flies. When you have taken enough, generally from a pint to a pint and a half from a strong grown person, untie the bandage and take it off, then double a small piece of linen rag into four, and put it on the cut; tie the bandage round the arm, over this rag, not too tight.

EPIDEMIC CHOLERA.

THE symptoms and treatment of this disease may be given under three heads or periods, which are easily separable, and each of which requires the administration of remedies properly adapted to it:—

I. The first stage (called by some *premonitory*) consists in most cases of a diarrhœa or bowel complaint of more or less intensity. Sometimes a degree of languor, sometimes nausea accompanies this condition of the bowels, attended by a sense of general uneasiness and discomfort. In many cases, however, the diarrhœa is the sole symptom. After the contents of the bowels have been evacuated, the discharges becomes thin and watery, and most commonly very copious. This condition of the patient varies from a few hours to three or four days; and can in almost every instance be arrested by the administration of ten or fifteen drops of laudanum, with the same quantity of spirits of camphor in two or three tablespoonfuls of water. The dose may be repeated every half hour or every hour (according to the urgency of the symptoms) until relief be obtained. When much languor or depression is present, the addition of from a half to one teaspoonful of tincture of red-pepper, compound spirits of lavender, tincture of ginger or tincture of cardamom, or ten or fifteen drops of the aromatic spirits of hartshorn, will be found very serviceable. Should the means just indicated fail, one of the following powders may be given at an interval of one or two hours according to circumstances: calomel two to five grains, sugar of lead from a half to one or two grains; or one of the following pills, at the interval indicated above:

18

sugar of lead one to two grains, powdered opium half to one grain. In connexion with these means, hot mustard poultices must be applied to the belly, and *absolute rest* enjoined. The diet should consist of arrowroot or rice gruel.

II. The second stage of the disease is characterized by oppressive nausea and vomiting; the matter thrown from the stomach being thin and watery. Violent cramps ensue, first of the stomach and intestines, and afterward of the muscles of the body and limbs, especially the latter. The evacuations are large and frequent. The patient very soon sinks into a state of collapse; the body becomes cold and clammy; the tongue pale and cold to the touch; the skin especially about the fingers wrinkled and sodden, as if the parts had been soaked in water; the countenance pale and sunken; the pulse which has been gradually becoming more and more feeble, is now scarcely perceptible; and the voice is hoarse, husky, and whispering. In this condition of things, all efforts must be directed to the re-establishment of warmth over the surface, and as prompt a return as possible to the healthy secretions of the body. To effect the first: hot mustard poultices with prompt and assiduous frictions with dry mustard, cayenne pepper or any stimulating liniment, or the application of hot air to the surface, should be commenced immediately. Bottles or tin cans containing hot water, bags of hot salt, ashes, &c., should be assiduously applied about the body and limbs. To effect the second result: internal stimulants, with or without opiates, according to the condition of the patient, should be carefully administered. The following recipe has well served this purpose :—

40 grains of calomel,
30 grains of best cayenne pepper,
15 grains of camphor,
10 grains of powdered opium ;

make into twenty pills; one of which may be given from every half hour to every two or three hours according to circumstances.

III. The third stage, that of reaction from this state of collapse resembles very strongly, with some modifications, an attack of mild typhus fever. As the frequent anomalies, however, which are exhibited, can not well be given in detail, it is impossible to offer any special treatment which would be generally applicable.

When the disease attacks suddenly after a full meal (which it sometimes does, the patient being suddenly seized with violent and excruciating cramps), the exhibition of some prompt emetic is absolutely necessary. The following will answer all the purposes required, viz.: one tablespoonful of common salt, and a good teaspoonful of strong mustard carefully rubbed up in a half tumbler of warm water. This dose may be repeated in the course of ten or fifteen minutes if necessary. After the stomach has thus been evacuated, the means indicated above may then be pursued, as the condition of the patient may demand.

Nothing has been said in reference to bleeding, because no general directions on this point can be made applicable. A physician must judge of the necessity before the remedy should be employed.

Under the head of preventives, nothing is of so much consequence as general and individual cleanliness, combined with a simple wholesome diet. Should the disease break out upon a plantation or appear in its neighborhood, a general purification should be *rigidly insisted* upon; and immediately upon the occurrence of the first case, a strict system of isolation should be at once commenced and continued during the prevalence of the disease.

GENERAL DIRECTIONS FOR RAISING NEGROES.

On every plantation great care should be taken in the building of negro-houses. The ground on which negro-houses are to be built should be raised higher in the middle, to allow the water to run off, for negroes will throw slops about them. If the spot is low, it should be well drained. Every house ought to be raised on blocks, or pillars, at least three feet from the ground, to allow the air to circulate under them freely and to avoid dampness. The floors should be tight, not only to prevent cold wind from affecting them, while asleep, but to prevent them from pouring slops through the floor; which, in my opinion, frequently gives rise to typhus fever. Every house should have a good chimney, for negroes sleep as often by the fire as in their beds. Some believe that smoke is wholesome. I do not deny it; but if a patient is sick, particularly with any complaint of the chest, as pleurisy or pneumonia, breathing an atmosphere filled with smoke is exceedingly injurious, and frequently fatal, as I have experienced.

One sleeping room, at least, in every house, should have a seat with a hole and cover, for the calls of nature ; because there are seldom or never any conveniences in the way of chambers ; and if they had them, they would immediately break them.   It is almost a universal practice among negroes to go into the open air for the calls of nature, in all kinds of weather.   This may answer when they are well, but in sickness they require more comfort.   I have known several cases of relapses which proved fatal, only because the patient was taking medicine, and was compelled to relieve himself in the open air, in the most inclement weather.   Planters can not attend to these little matters always, and plantation nurses generally will not.

On every plantation, also, there should be a capable and trusty nurse, to attend the sick and to report all new cases. A faithful and trusty woman (not as is commonly the case, a decrepit old woman), but a strong, able, and healthy woman to attend the negro children ; for mothers who have infants at the breast will frequently obtain leave of absence from the field to nurse their infants and employ the time given them in sleeping.

The person selected for the little negroes should also be made to cook for them, and to see that they are fed regularly with victuals well cooked.   For it is a common practice among negroes to eat victuals half raw, and of course to give the same to their children.   Some do it from laziness, others from ignorance of cooking, and some leave the feeding of their children entirely to their little nurses.   I have several times been called to attend little children on plantations, who were poor and emaciated, and as the planter or overseer termed it, *not thriving*, but who were evidently suffering actually from starvation and want of water, owing to the negligence of their parents and little nurses.   Now a planter who would make such a regulation as to insure each child having two meals well cooked, a day, and which, even on a large plantation could be performed by one person cooking for all at once, in one large, or two or three cooking utensils, would, in my opinion, be richly repaid, not only by the number of children raised, but he would positively save in provisions ; for it is a common thing for negroes to keep their week's allowance of provisions carelessly emptied on a shelf, or table, in their houses, exposed to rats, fowls, and to general waste. Their salt is kept in the same way, and it is evident that they or their children, who are so improvident, must frequently suffer, or the loss must be made up by stealing from the others. Now it is evident that the average of a peck of corn a week, to each grown negro, is ample allowance, for with all their waste, some raise several fowls and hogs, and few are without a dog. It is an old custom to give each negro their allowance, and no doubt the provident save the surplus, and with the proceeds, either sold or bartered, procure many comforts. But I believe that if the experiment was generally made of having the food of the grown negroes all cooked together, and meals served to each regularly, it would not only be more satisfactory to the negroes themselves, generally, but the planter would be enabled by what he saved in provisions, to give them many a meal of bacon, than which no food is more palatable or wholesome for a negro. The negroes, also, would be more healthy, for they would eat at least two meals well cooked, during the day, and be, in a measure, prevented from sitting up and gourmandizing at night, a practice which is very common, and seldom fails to induce indigestion, diarrhœa, and constant indisposition.

The use of bacon, also, is a great preventive of indigestion, for the grease acting mechanically on the bowels, causes the food, even if half cooked, to pass through the bowels more easily and quickly.

It has been observed, that in all countries where the working-classes use olive oil (and among most of them the food is worse than that of our negroes), diseases from indigestion, such as dyspepsia, cholera-morbus, diarrhœa, dysentery, &c., with which our negroes are constantly affected, very seldom occur. It is a notorious fact, also, that in all countries, the peasantry who are much more exposed, and work much harder than our negroes, nevertheless increase rapidly, and raise a great many children, while the reverse takes place on our plantations. And I sincerely believe that it is owing to the causes which I have mentioned, and the planter who wishes his negroes to be healthy, must not allow them to indulge their natural propensities. In Africa, in their free state, they are among the most barbarous inhabitants of the earth, living in the woods and subsisting chiefly on the natural productions of the earth. They retain their habits and propensities the same among us, and we must not expect to find among them the same providence or civilization as is observed among the poorest classes in Europe. I have known plantations on which the increase of the negroes bore a fair proportion to the crop, and made up the losses of them, and where planters, working poor lands, thus kept pace with those planting the best, and even surpassed them. In one case, ten infants were born the same year, and all raised, and no death occurred on this place for three years, except one from old age. The regulations here were such as I have recommended, and strict attention paid to the cleanliness of the negroes, and a punishment inflicted on all who were seen ragged and dirty. I have observed that those negroes who were the most filthy in their persons, were generally, also, the most unhealthy, and many diseases of the skin which are supposed to be scrofula, and treated as such, arise entirely from filth of the body.

Planters should also supply their negroes with combs, and enforce the use of them daily. Many of the eruptions which appear to be diseases of the scalp, are caused entirely by vermin, and consequent scratching. Finally; I am convinced that if more system and discipline (like regulations in an army), were pursued on plantations, the condition of the negroes, as well as that of the planter, would be materially improved, and the per-centage of the latter, which seldom reaches, or at least exceeds, in the course of years, seven per-cent. on his investment, would be much increased, as also the condition of our entire population at the south rendered more flourishing, all classes of which, professions and trades, are affected, more or less, by the success or failure of the planter.

THE END.

CPSIA information can be obtained at www.ICGtesting.com
Printed in the USA
244045LV00001B/1/P